21 Habits

A Wellness Survival Guide

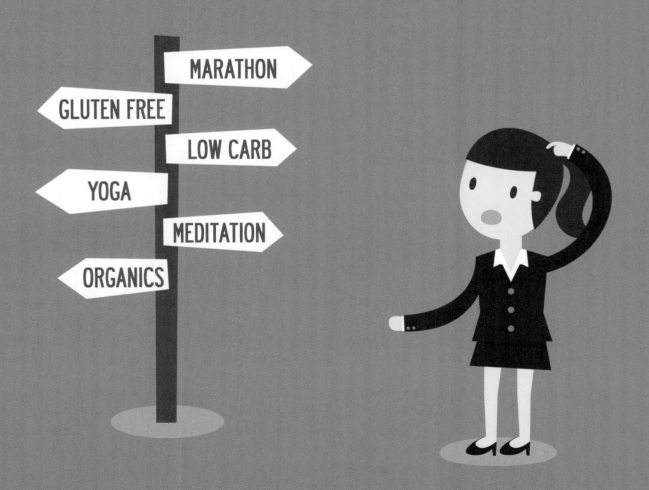

MARATHON

GLUTEN FREE

LOW CARB

YOGA

MEDITATION

ORGANICS

Michael Guercio and Tad Mitchell

Thank you to Tad for giving me an opportunity to help others while challenging me to think further outside of the box. Thank you to Renee, Pamela, and Tricia, our editing extraordinaires. Thank you to Doug for your brilliance and artistic vision. A sincere thank you to all of our reviewers for leaving no stone unturned. And a special thank you to my wife and kids for their optimism, patience, and unwavering support.

Michael

Thank you to Michael who patiently educated me in wellness and endured several major directional changes. Thank you to our editors: Renee, Pamela, and Tricia. Thank you to our reviewers. Thank you to Doug who tirelessly worked on iterating the artwork until it was right and did the layout with his special eye for precision. Thank you to all who provided feedback, especially my wife, France, who put all her heart into making this a wonderful product.

Tad

Dedicated to the healthy person inside of everyone.

Contents

How to Build a Habit

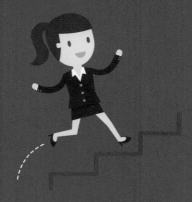

1. Believe It
2. Shrink It
3. Trigger It
4. Prepare for It
5. Track It
6. Be It

The 21 Habits

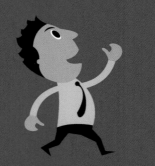

1. Eat just enough
2. Drink enough water
3. Sleep enough
4. Enjoy fruits and vegetables daily
5. Enjoy beans
6. Enjoy whole grains
7. Enjoy sunshine in moderation
8. Enjoy fats in moderation
9. Enjoy meat in moderation
10. Enjoy dairy in moderation
11. Limit alcohol
12. Limit caffeine
13. Limit sugar
14. Limit deep-fried foods
15. Forgo tobacco
16. Move
17. Strengthen
18. Stretch
19. Be positive
20. Socialize daily
21. Recharge daily

Recipicks

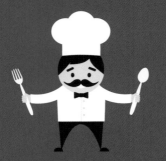

1. Vegetable Soup
2. Stir Fry
3. Fruit Salad
4. Smoothie
5. Beans and Rice
6. Bean Salad
7. Hummus
8. Vinaigrette
9. Mayonnaise

Foreword

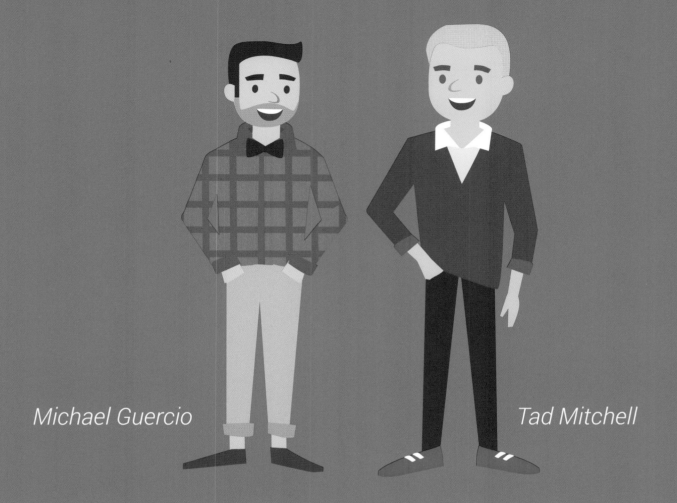

Michael Guercio   Tad Mitchell

In today's world, there is so much information about being healthy that it's hard to know where to begin. *21 Habits* cuts to the core of healthy living, explains exactly where to begin, and gives practical tips on how to succeed. But the best part of *21 Habits* isn't about health at all. It's about transforming yourself through habits. While habits seem quite simple, they're more complex than you think. *21 Habits* will help you successfully add new habits to your life and become the best version of yourself.

We hope you enjoy the simple beauty of *21 Habits*. It's changed our lives for good, and we hope that it will do the same for you.

How to
Build a Habit

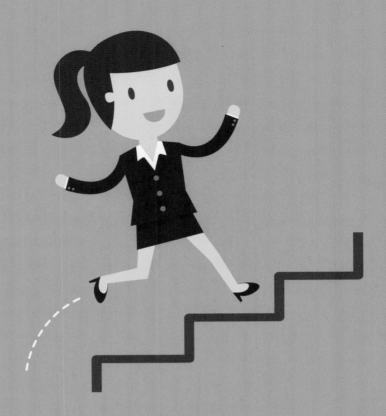

You are the sum of your habits. Thus, the only way to change yourself is to change your habits.
Initially, it takes some focus and work to build a habit, but once you build a habit (or break a
habit), your mind is free to work on something else. You have literally rewired your brain to do a
new routine without even thinking. That is the power of habits.

Wellness is similar. Your health is the sum of your wellness habits. You can go on a diet or
start an exercise routine in hopes of losing some weight, but unless you build new habits in the
process, you will eventually revert to your previous wellness level. By focusing on small habits,
you can change your wellness level and your life for good.

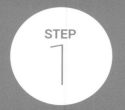

STEP
1

Believe It

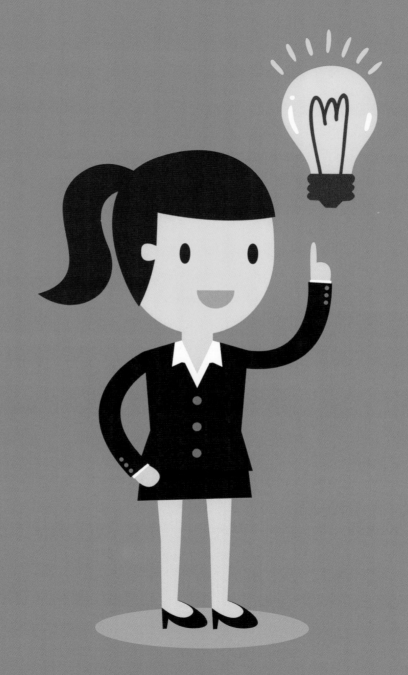

Pick a habit that you are excited about and believe in. If you are not completely convinced that you want a particular habit, then it's much harder to master it. Study the habit, think about why it may be important, and let the desire to change grow within you. Forming and sticking to a new habit is much easier if you are sold on it.

A good test to see if you really believe in a habit is to ask yourself if you are ready to keep that habit for the rest of your life. If you aren't, you're probably trying to shortcut the process, which will end up giving you a short-lived result. Slow and steady wins the race. You'll be more successful over time if you build smaller habits that you actually intend to do for the rest of your life.

Tips

- **Trust your gut.** Pick a habit that you feel good about. Don't work on a habit because someone else thinks it's a good idea. Remember this is your journey, not someone else's.

- **Educate yourself.** Take time to learn firsthand about why the habit is important. Talk with others about their experiences before and after they mastered the habit.

- **Try again.** Pick a habit that you've previously mastered and then fallen away from. Before you try again, take time to reflect on why this habit did not stick, learn more about why this habit is important, and make sure you truly believe in it before you try again.

- **Coach yourself.** Speak to yourself positively. Tell yourself that you can do it and that you can be successful at what you choose to do. You will become the person you believe you are.

- **Visualize it.** Picture in your mind what you will be like after implementing the habit for 1 week; 1 month; 5 years. Visualization helps you become the person you want to be.

- **Do a 30-day trial.** If you really want to build a habit but aren't sure if you can do it over the long-term, do a 30-day trial. After your trial, you can reevaluate if the habit is right for you.

Shrink It

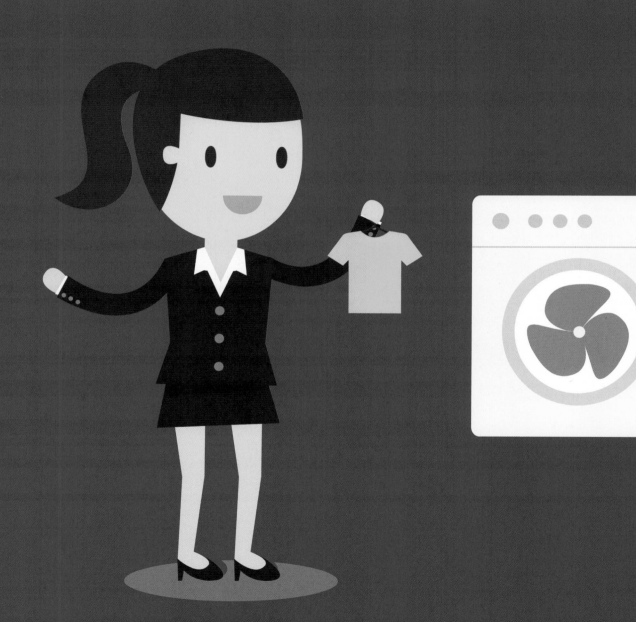

Pick a habit that is small and easy. If you want to eat more vegetables, start by eating just one vegetable a day. If you end up eating more than one vegetable some days, great! The important thing is to keep your expectations small until this habit becomes ingrained. Once you have mastered this habit, you can certainly expand it to eating plenty of veggies every day. Starting small can be liberating because it's so simple and doable.

Only work on one habit at a time. As tempting as it is to try to change everything at once, if you try to develop more than one new habit at a time, you decrease your chances of success.

Tips

- **Pick a daily habit.** Pick a habit that you can do each day. Daily habits are typically smaller, repetitive habits that produce big changes over time.

- **Aim low.** Set your goals low. If you think you might be able to do 50 push-ups a day but know for sure that you can do 20 push-ups a day, start with 20 push-ups. If you do more than 20, great! But if you only do 20, you've still succeeded.

- **Set a time range.** If your habit requires you to do something all day long (not drinking coffee), start working within a small time range (no coffee after 2 PM) and expand the range over time.

- **Break it down.** Write your habit at the top of a piece of paper. Use a tree structure to keep breaking your habit into smaller and smaller habits. Choose one of the smallest habits to work on first.

- **Allow for exceptions.** Set rules for when and how much you will cheat. For example, I will only eat french fries once a week or I will only eat dessert with Sunday dinner. Cheats can turn an impossible habit into a lifestyle that you can maintain for a lifetime. Rules make it easy because then you don't need to decide each time. Cheats also alleviate the guilt from those occasions when you'd like to indulge, which can make you want to give up on your habit completely.

STEP
3

Trigger It

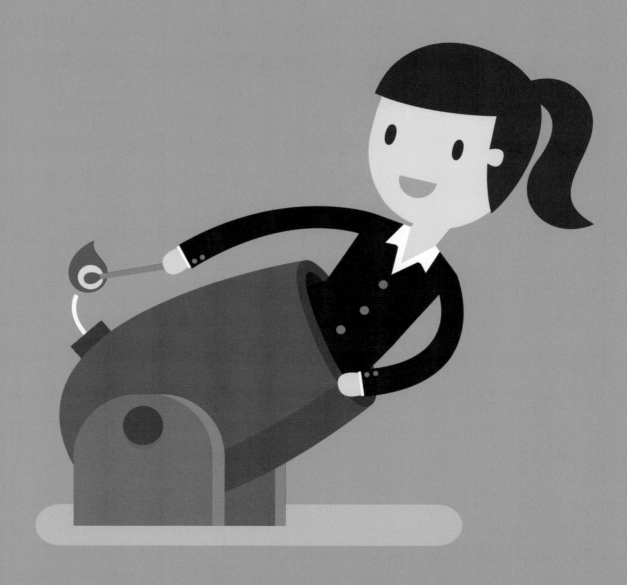

A trigger is something that sparks a behavior. You may not even realize this happens, but you have triggers that cause you to do things all day long. To start a new habit, you need to find a good trigger to initiate the habit. The best triggers are things that already happen every day. Getting ready to leave your home is a trigger. Every time you leave home, you can fill up a water bottle. Filling up the water bottle becomes the new habit. Simply seeing the water bottle can be another trigger to prompt you to drink more water.

Tips

- **Set a time.** Establish a specific time and day(s) that you will do your habit. Simply knowing what time you are going to do it may be enough. If not, set a recurring alarm so you'll never forget.

- **Use a natural trigger.** Use something that already happens in your life as the trigger. When you go to bed, read a book. After you eat dinner, take a walk.

- **Invite a friend.** Inviting a friend to do a habit with you is a very powerful trigger. Not only does it trigger you to do your habit, it holds you accountable.

- **Use a visual trigger.** Put a note on the wall or put something in a specific place to remind yourself. Put a note on the fridge to remind yourself to make your lunch. Put the floss on the counter next to your toothbrush to remind yourself to floss.

- **Change it up.** If you are having a hard time with a habit, it may be the trigger, not the habit. Choose a different trigger and try again. Say you've decided to do 15 push-ups every hour on the hour for a break, but you keep forgetting because you get wrapped up in your work. Try using going to the bathroom as your trigger instead. Since this forces you to get up, it may be a more effective trigger.

Breaking Bad Habits: You can break a bad habit by removing what triggers the habit or by replacing the bad habit with a good habit. For example, if you want to stop eating pastries in the morning, change your morning route so you don't drive by the pastry shop. If you like drinking soda in the late afternoon when you feel tired, take a five-minute walk instead. Identifying the trigger for a habit you want to give up is key to replacing it with a new habit.

Prepare for It

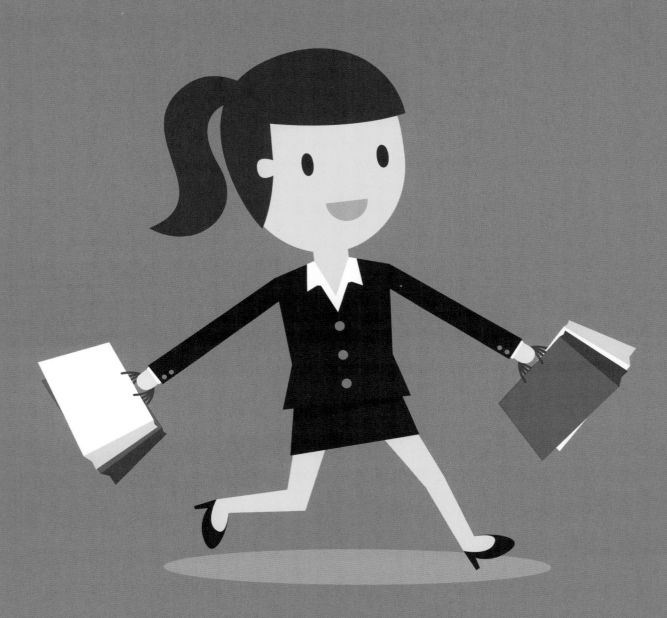

You would never go on a trip without preparing for it. Building a new habit is similar. If you are not prepared, your journey will be much less enjoyable, and you may not even make it to your destination. Being prepared for your journey can make all the difference.

Tips

- **Go shopping.** For many habits, you need to make a shopping list and go to the store before you start. If you are going to start eating more whole grains, shop around to find the place that makes the best whole-wheat bread. If you are going to write in a journal, buy yourself a nice journal or notebook.

- **Clean house.** You may need to change your environment to be successful. If you are going to try to stop snacking, get the snacks out of your cupboards. If you are going to start meditating, prepare a nice, relaxing place in your home where you can meditate.

- **Research.** Spend time learning about what you will be doing before you do it. If you are going to start cooking more, choose recipes you will try. If you want to take more time to recharge, research places where you can go on the weekend.

- **Plan.** Make sure you have allocated enough time for your new habit. If you are going to start painting, schedule specific days and times for painting. Decide what you will paint first. If you are going to start cooking more, make sure you plan ahead for days when you won't have enough time to cook. Plan a simple meal or plan to eat leftovers.

- **Plan for obstacles.** Life will get in your way. Birthday parties and vacations will happen. Don't let them knock you off track. Instead, think ahead and put a plan in place. Decide that you will have a piece of cake, but that's all. Better yet, create a way to redeem yourself. Decide that you will walk an extra 30 minutes every time you fall short.

- **Plan to restart.** Make a plan for how you will restart when you get off track. If weekends are challenging, have a plan in place to start strong every Monday.

Track It

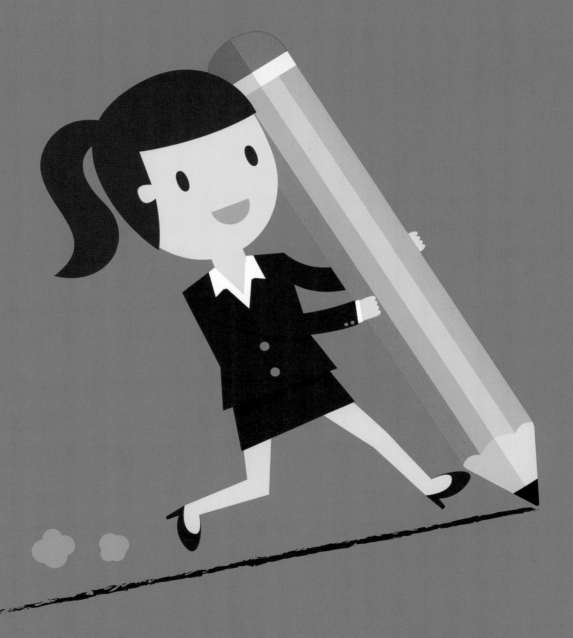

Each time you work on creating a new habit, track it. It will help you see your progress as you go. Building a habit can take a while, so be patient with yourself. Some habits can be formed in a few weeks. Others might take months. Just keep working on it until you feel confident that it has become part of your regular routine. If you stop for some reason, start again. Your next attempt will be more successful.

Tips

- **Mark your calendar.** Place a mark on your calendar each day when you have succeeded with your habit. Seeing your progress over time can inspire you to keep going.

- **Keep a tally.** Keep a piece of paper on your desk or reserve part of your whiteboard to keep a tally. It will serve as a visual reminder and a reward each time you do your habit.

- **Tell your friends.** Tell one or more friends what you are doing. Talk to them about your experiences. Pretty soon they'll start asking you how it is going.

- **Report to a friend.** Ask a friend if you can report your results to them periodically. This approach makes you accountable and gives you some support.

- **Mark your planner.** If you keep a daily planner, track your progress there.

- **Celebrate milestones.** Plan to reward yourself as you reach predetermined goals. Use positive rewards like new running shoes or a vacation.

Be It

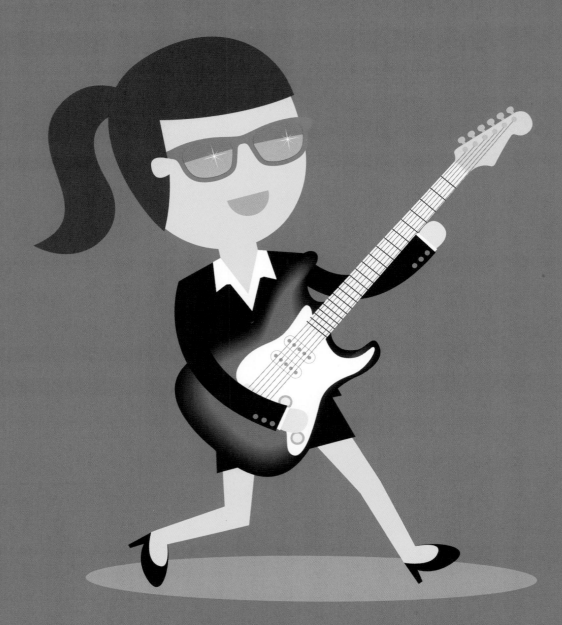

In order for you to keep doing your new habit for the rest of your life, it needs to become ingrained as part of your identity, of who you are. If you stop eating donuts, to keep it up over the long term, you need to believe you are a healthy person, the type of person that rarely eats a donut. A habit is never a habit for life until it becomes part of who you are.

Tips

- **Tell your friends.** Share your new habits with your friends. If you tell your friends that you no longer drink soda, they'll support you and won't let you drink soda even if you try.

- **Make new friends.** If you quit smoking, you may need to find new friends who don't smoke. Other habits can be similar. You may need to make new friends that share your new, healthy lifestyle.

- **Accept your new self.** If someone points out that you always go to the gym or you don't eat french fries, don't dispute them. Accept these statements as part of who you are.

- **Buy new clothes.** If you've lost weight, buy new clothes that fit you and give your old clothes to charity. Believe that you will never go back to your old self.

- **Create a motto.** Come up with a motto like "I'm a clean machine" to remind yourself of what you stand for. Repeat your motto when you're faced with tough decisions.

- **Build on your strengths.** Continue to build habits in areas in which you are naturally strong. If you like to be active, work on your fitness habits first. If cooking is your thing, start by trying some new, healthy recipes. Building on your existing identity is much easier than building a new one.

The 21 Habits

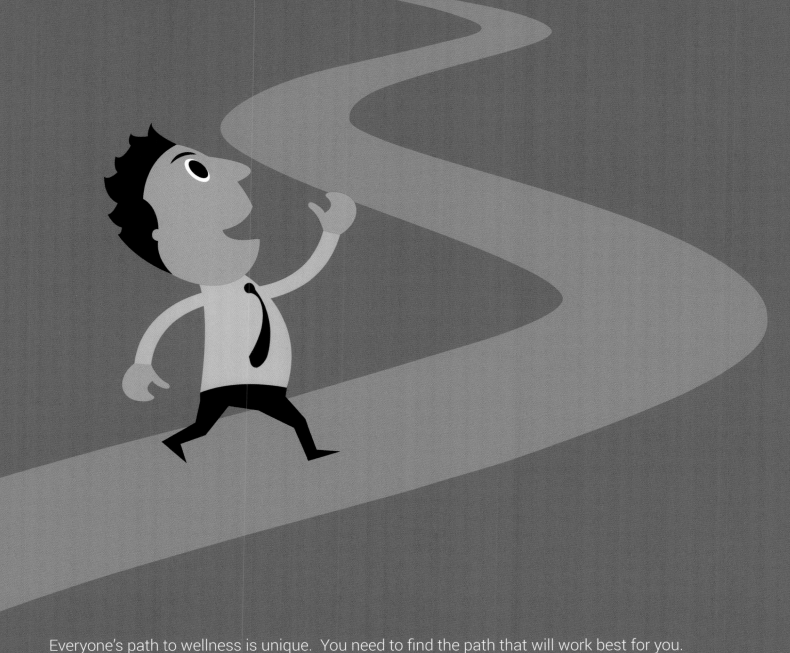

Everyone's path to wellness is unique. You need to find the path that will work best for you. Pick a habit that you believe in, and work on it until you have mastered it. Keep repeating this process day by day, week after week, for the rest of your life, and you will go places you never imagined. Strive for progress, not perfection, and enjoy your journey. Along the way, you will find much more than wellness.

Eat just enough

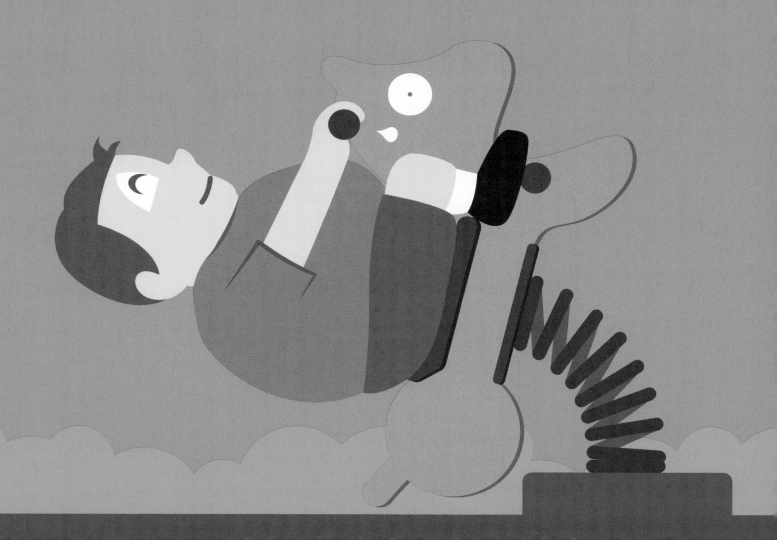

You're probably laughing out loud right now thinking, "Eat just enough? I wish it were that simple." Obviously, it's not. For most people, eating just enough food is their biggest struggle with wellness, not whether they exercise enough. A half-hour workout (300 calories) can quickly be erased by a burger (500 calories), fries (400 calories), and drink (200 calories). Also, with exercise, you only need to make one decision each day. With food, you need to make dozens of decisions throughout the day. This is why 14 of the 21 Habits are dedicated to food.

Even though it's tough, not overeating is extremely important since obesity rivals smoking for the highest cause of premature deaths.[1] Don't despair. Just focus on one habit at a time, and you will get there. The Small Habits below help you eat less. The rest of the Habits in the book help you eat healthier foods, exercise, and build your mental strength. You can do it!

Small Habits

- ☐ **Weigh yourself monthly.** Track your weight (or body measurements) like the stock market. Expect ups and downs but see what the overall picture is telling you.

- ☐ **Eat slowly.** Take the time to savor your food and the company of those around you. This gives your stomach the 15-20 minutes it needs to tell your brain it's full.

- ☐ **Dine.** Eat at the dining table. When you eat in front of the television, your desk, or on the go, it is far too easy to overeat because you are not focused on the fact that you're eating.

- ☐ **Skip seconds.** Serve yourself reasonable portions, and then don't go back for more. Put food away and out of sight after serving to help avoid the temptation.

- ☐ **Split a meal.** When dining out, split a meal with a friend or put half of the meal in a to-go container before you start to eat.

- ☐ **Close the kitchen.** After dinner, clean up the kitchen, turn out the lights, and don't go back in for the rest of the evening.

- ☐ **Don't eat out of the bag.** Instead of eating out of the bag or box, pour some in a bowl so you know how much you are eating.

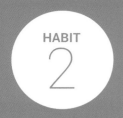

HABIT
2

Drink enough water

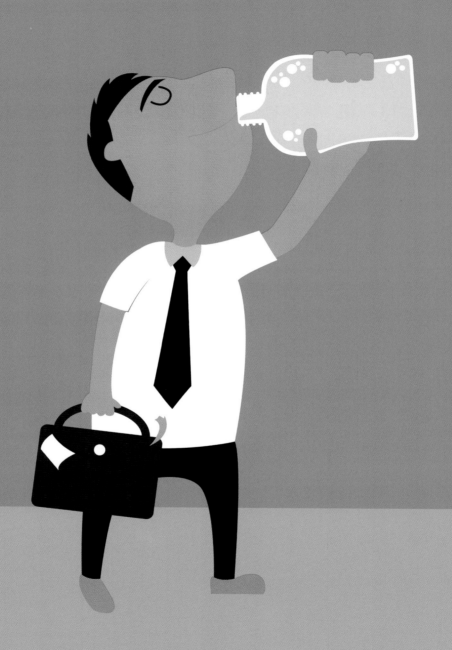

With all the talk about drinking water lately, you might wonder if you are drinking enough water and why it's so important in the first place. It's true that being properly hydrated is important, but it's not that complicated. If you are thirsty, you should drink something. Water is your best choice, but other drinks will hydrate you as well. If you urinate less than every 4 to 5 hours, drink more.

Water is needed for almost every aspect of your body to work well. When you are hot, perspiration cools you down. Your blood (which is mostly water) brings nutrients to your body and collects waste. Your kidneys filter the blood, producing urine. Water keeps your stools soft (less constipation) and lubricates your joints (less pain and injury). Proper hydration even helps you think clearly[2] and may lessen the duration and intensity of headaches.[3]

Small Habits

- ☐ **Substitute water.** Drink water instead of your normal beverage one or more times a day.
- ☐ **Keep water handy.** Bring a water bottle with you wherever you go or keep a glass of water at your desk. As soon as you hit the bottom, refill it right away.
- ☐ **Wake up to water.** Start the day off with a glass of water.
- ☐ **Add some zest.** Try adding fresh lemon juice, mint leaves, sliced strawberries, or cut cucumber to your water bottle in the morning.
- ☐ **Dine with water.** When dining, choose water to accompany your meal to reduce overall calorie intake.

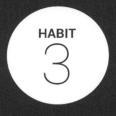

HABIT
3

Sleep enough

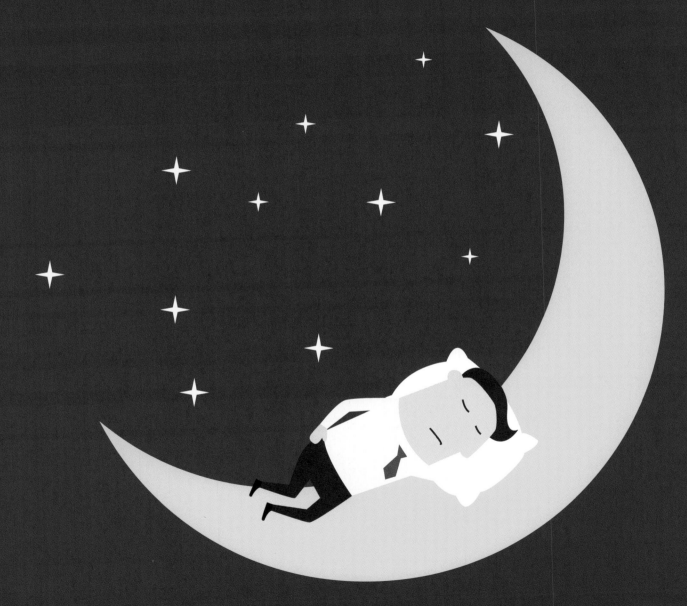

In today's busy world, getting enough sleep is a luxury most people only get to enjoy on the weekend, if then. There just aren't enough hours in the day. Still, it's important to understand the benefits of sleep and strive towards getting the optimal amount. As little as 15 to 30 minutes more a day can help. Even if you can't find more time, better sleep practices can help you sleep more deeply and wake up feeling more refreshed.

Sleeping strengthens your immune system, helps you solve problems, helps you reason better, and increases your memory.[4] Getting the right amount of sleep can make you happier and less irritable throughout the day. Proper sleep even makes it easier for you to control your weight.[5]

Age	Sleep requirement
0 to 3 months	14 to 17 hours
4 months to 5 years	11 to 15 hours
6 to 17 years	9 to 11 hours
18 years and older	7 to 9 hours

Source: National Sleep Foundation.

Small Habits

- ☐ **Keep a bedtime routine.** Do the same series of activities leading up to bedtime (put on your pajamas, brush your teeth, read a book, go to sleep). Keep a consistent bedtime.

- ☐ **Prepare your bedroom.** Make sure your bed is comfortable, and the room is dark and quiet. Reducing the temperature in your bedroom can help too.

- ☐ **Prevent interruptions.** Stop drinking fluids at least 90 minutes before bedtime. Silence your cell phone.

- ☐ **Avoid caffeine, alcohol, and tobacco.** Do not consume any caffeine in the afternoon or evening. Avoid alcohol and tobacco late in the evening.

- ☐ **Shut down the media.** Do not use any media (TV, computer, cell phone) for an hour before going to bed because the blue light emitted from these devices mimics daylight, telling your brain it is time to be awake.[6]

- ☐ **Clear your mind.** If your mind starts to wander, use your breath as an anchor to the present, restful moment.

- ☐ **Don't eat late at night.** Eating before bedtime can reduce the quality of your sleep.[7]

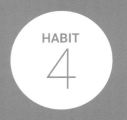

Enjoy fruits and vegetables daily

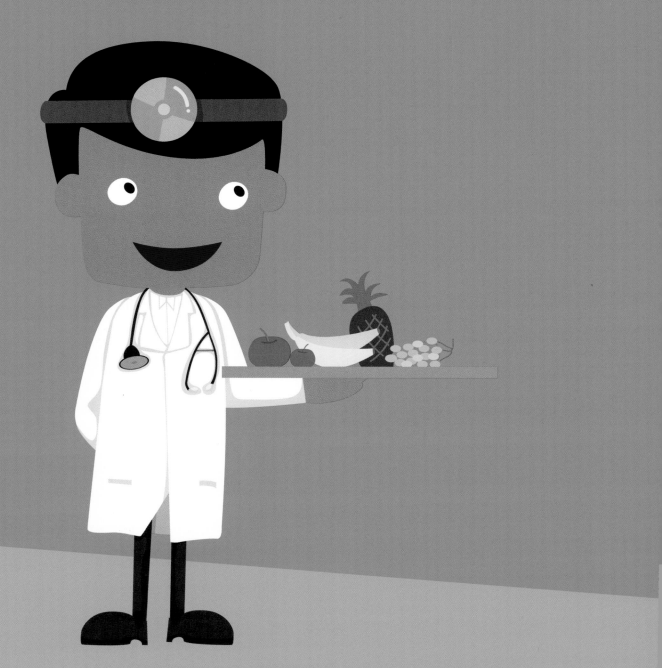

Eating five fruits or vegetables a day is a stretch for most people, because that is quite a lot. While you may never be a five-a-day person, eating just one more than you usually eat each day can make a big impact on your health.

Fruits and vegetables help protect the body from illness and disease. When you eat several different plants together, their effects are magnified. For example, when broccoli and tomatoes are eaten together, the effect is even more potent.[8] Be sure to eat a variety of fruits and vegetables because each one has its own special properties. Also, alternate eating them cooked and raw. Cooking destroys some nutrients while making others more available.

Small Habits

- ☐ **Enjoy salad.** Eat salad as an entrée or side for lunch or dinner. Be creative. Try coleslaw, cucumber salad, beet salad, tomato salad, shredded carrot salad, or any creation that sounds good to you.

- ☐ **Enjoy vegetable soup.** Start your dinner with vegetable soup. It is low in calories and fills you up. It's also easy to hide vegetables that your family would not normally eat if you purée the soup. (See *Recipicks*.)

- ☐ **Fill half your plate with vegetables.** Consciously fill half of the space on your plate with vegetables. This naturally decreases the total amount of calories in your meal.

- ☐ **Have a smoothie.** Start your day with a smoothie. Smoothies are a great way to increase your fruit and vegetable intake, and it's easy to get five servings in a single smoothie. (See *Recipicks*.)

- ☐ **Enjoy fruit at breakfast.** Eating fruit at breakfast is a great way to start the day. Fruit is tasty plain, or you can mix it with yogurt, cottage cheese, nuts, or cereal.

- ☐ **Enjoy fruit for dessert.** Satisfy your sweet tooth with fruit. To make it feel more like dessert, make a fruit salad or fruit platter or serve it in a dessert cup with a sprig of mint.

- ☐ **Make fruits and vegetables visible.** Increase your chance of picking a healthy snack by displaying fruits on your kitchen counter and leaving prepared veggies on the main shelf in your fridge. If you see them, you will eat them.

HABIT
5

Enjoy beans

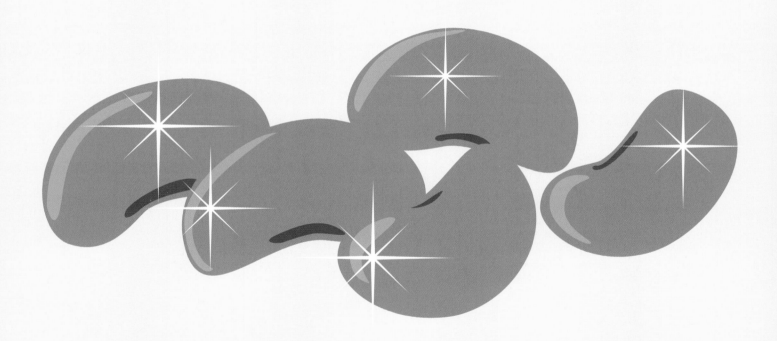

If you're like most people, the last time you ate beans was at a summer barbecue, and the thought of eating beans every day seems ridiculous (unless you're from a culture that naturally does so). The reality is you'll probably never eat beans every day. Just try to eat them more often. Even if you only eat them once a week or once a month, you'll be healthier for it.

Beans are packed with nutrients and are a great source of protein and fiber. Fiber improves digestion, helps remove toxins from your body, and even slightly reduces your cholesterol.[9] Fiber is so beneficial that it reduces your chance of disease by 10% for every 10 grams you eat each day.[10] Eating beans also helps you live longer.[11]

Small Habits

- ☐ **Enjoy beans and rice weekly.** Find some beans and rice recipes that you like and add them to your cooking repertoire. Many cultures eat beans and rice daily.

- ☐ **Enjoy a side of beans weekly.** Use beans as a side dish for dinner at least once a week. Pork and beans are easy to warm and serve. Check the international aisle in the grocery store for other ready-to-serve bean dishes.

- ☐ **Substitute hummus.** Try hummus instead of dip with vegetables or pita bread. Use hummus as the "meat" on your sandwich. (See *Recipicks*.)

- ☐ **Enjoy beans with grains.** When combined with grains, beans provide a complete protein.

- ☐ **Keep bean salad in the fridge.** Purchase or make a bean salad and keep it in the fridge. Most bean salads will keep for a week or more and make a great side for any meal.

Bean Cooking Tips

- **Reduce gas.** Soak dry beans 12 to 24 hours prior to cooking then discard the water to greatly reduce the compound (raffinose), which is known to cause gas. Rinse canned beans prior to use to achieve the same results.
- **Use a pressure cooker.** A pressure cooker can dramatically reduce the cooking time for beans.
- **Try lentils.** Lentils cook much faster than beans, don't require soaking, and provide all the same benefits.
- **Freeze bean dishes.** Since bean dishes can take a long time to prepare, make a large batch and freeze some for another day.

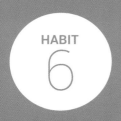

HABIT
6

Enjoy whole grains

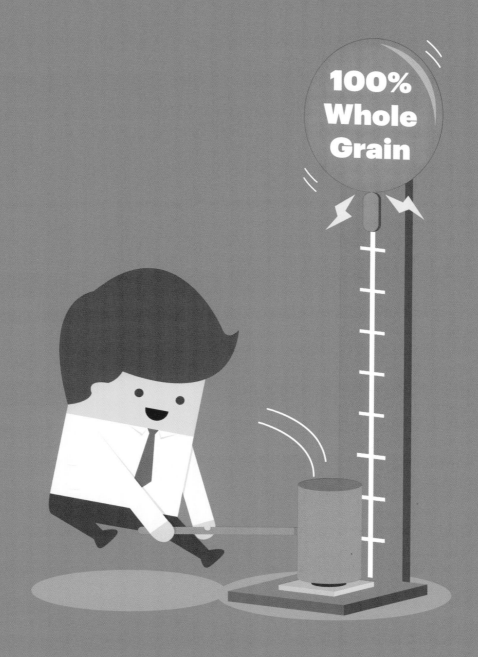

100%
Whole
Grain

Remember the days when bread and rice were considered healthy and wholesome? What happened? Now carbs are seen as the enemy, even whole grains. Everyone seems to be on a diet that limits grains. Despite these recent trends, grains are still just as nutritious as fruits, vegetables, and beans.[12] The trick is you need to eat *whole* grains, not *refined* grains. Refined grains (white flour, white bread, white rice, and pasta) have had the nutritious parts (the bran and the germ) removed, leaving only the calorie-dense, starchy center. Make sure you don't go overboard. Whole grains are good for you, but one serving per meal is plenty.

Small Habits

- **Enjoy 100% whole-grain bread.** Only buy products that are labeled "100% whole grain." Products labeled "wheat," "whole wheat," "multigrain," or "seven-grain," usually only contain 15%-50% whole grain.

- **Enjoy brown rice.** Use brown or wild rice instead of white rice. It has a wonderful nutty flavor.

- **Enjoy oatmeal.** Try oatmeal for breakfast. Quick, old-fashioned, and steel-cut oats are all whole grain and can be ready in minutes. Watch out for pre-sweetened packages, which contain large amounts of sugar. Instead, sweeten your oatmeal with fresh fruit, raisins, nuts, or honey.

- **Substitute popcorn.** Enjoy popcorn instead of chips. Pop your own to avoid additives. Try using coconut oil and sea salt.

- **Look twice at your dry cereal.** Choose an unsweetened cereal that has whole grain as the first ingredient. Most contain high amounts of sugar and little if any whole grain.

- **Try something new.** Try quinoa, millet, farro, polenta, and buckwheat. They each have unique textures and flavors. Most can be cooked like rice and served as a side dish.

Whole-Grain Cooking Tips

- **Use a rice cooker.** A rice cooker makes perfectly cooked rice. It can also be used to cook oatmeal, wheat, quinoa, and other ancient grains—even whole-grain pasta.
- **Freeze brown rice.** Since brown rice typically takes 45 minutes to cook instead of 20, you may want to cook extra and freeze it for a day when you are in a rush.
- **Use a pressure cooker.** A pressure cooker can cook brown rice and other grains in less than 20 minutes.

Enjoy sunshine in moderation

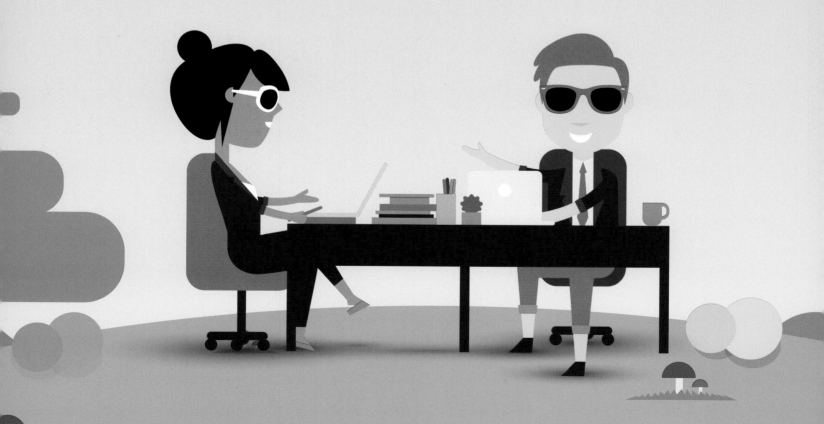

With the alarming possibility of getting skin cancer, you've probably been told to slather on the sunscreen every time you're out in the sun for an extended period. Good. That's what you should be doing. On the other extreme, if you don't get out in the sun enough, you may be deficient in vitamin D, which helps prevent sickness and disease, strengthen your bones,[13] and improve your mood.[14]

Your body creates vitamin D when sunshine contacts your skin. People with light skin can produce enough vitamin D in as little as 5-10 minutes with exposure to legs and arms 2-3 times per week.[15] People with darker skin require up to 8 times this exposure.[16] Even though you probably won't have any problem getting enough sunshine in the summer, the Small Habits below will help you boost your vitamin-D levels during the other seasons.

Small Habits

- ☐ **Take a walk.** Take a brief walk in the middle of the day to take advantage of the sun's rays when they are the strongest.

- ☐ **Eat lunch outside.** If it's a sunny day, eat lunch outside.

- ☐ **Roll up your sleeves.** When you are in the sun for brief periods of time, take off your jacket or roll up your sleeves to expose more skin and increase vitamin-D production.

- ☐ **Take a winter vacation.** Save your airline miles for a vacation in a warm, sunny place during the winter months. Since your body can store vitamin D for up to two months, a vacation in a warm place can do a lot to boost your body's vitamin-D supply.[17]

- ☐ **Consider a vitamin-D supplement.** Consult your physician about taking a vitamin-D3 supplement during the months you cannot get enough sunshine. Vitamin D3 is a fat-soluble vitamin and should be consumed with healthy fats.

- ☐ **Wear sunscreen when needed.** Use sunscreen when you will be in the sun for extended periods of time (hours).[18] Overexposure to the sun causes wrinkling, aging skin, and skin cancer.

- ☐ **Eat fish weekly.** Fatty fish (salmon, sardines, mackerel) is nature's best food source of vitamin D. Milk is fortified with vitamin D, but you need to drink three glasses a day.

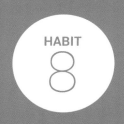

Enjoy fats in moderation

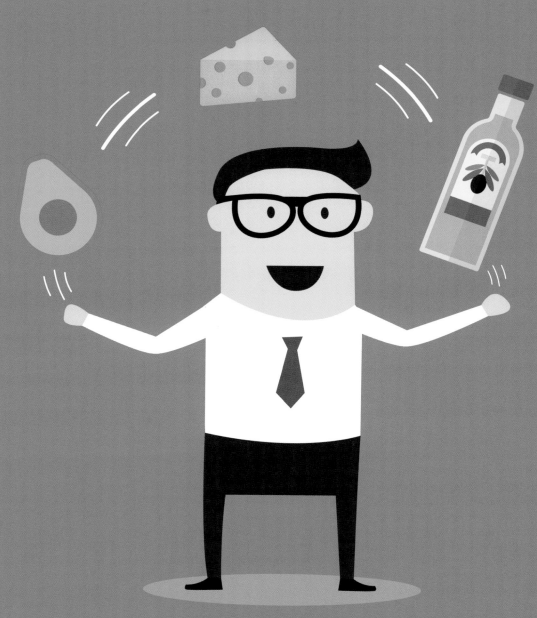

You probably already limit how much fat you eat to some degree. It stands to reason that fat makes you fat. Right? Not necessarily. It is true that fat has twice the calories of carbs and protein, but you can get fat eating too much of any food. In fact, you must include fat in your diet to be healthy. Fat is used to create the structure of your cells. Fat is also necessary for your body to absorb essential fat-soluble vitamins A, D, E, and K.

The best way to include fat in your diet is by eating a variety of whole foods that contain fat, like avocados, olives, nuts, seeds, eggs, milk, cheese, and meat. Oils, processed or not, should be used sparingly. Variety and moderation are key as each fat source has unique benefits and all are high in calories. Good fat is essential, but one source of fat per meal is plenty.

Small Habits

- ☐ **Enjoy nuts in moderation.** A handful of nuts can have 200 or more calories. Try buying nuts still in the shell to slow yourself down to the pace nature intended. Opt for unsalted nuts.

- ☐ **Avoid bad fats.** Hydrogenated and partially hydrogenated oils (trans fats: fry oil, shortening, and stick margarine) should be avoided as they have been shown to cause heart disease.[19]

- ☐ **Sauté with liquid.** Sauté with water, broth, or vinegar instead of oil.

- ☐ **Substitute applesauce.** When you bake, replace part or all of the butter or oil with applesauce in a 1:1 ratio. One half cup of butter has 800 calories while one half cup of applesauce has only 80 calories.

- ☐ **Choose extra virgin plant oils.** Use extra virgin plant oils (olive, avocado, flaxseed, sesame). Extra virgin means that the oil has not been refined with heat or chemicals. Just like whole grains, extra virgin oils contain more nutrients.

- ☐ **Make your own salad dressing.** Make your own salad dressing with virgin plant oil. It only takes a couple minutes, and it tastes better. (See *Recipicks*.)

- ☐ **Bake from scratch.** Store-bought baked goods and mixes are often made with hydrogenated oil. Take the time to bake your own treats with healthy oil.

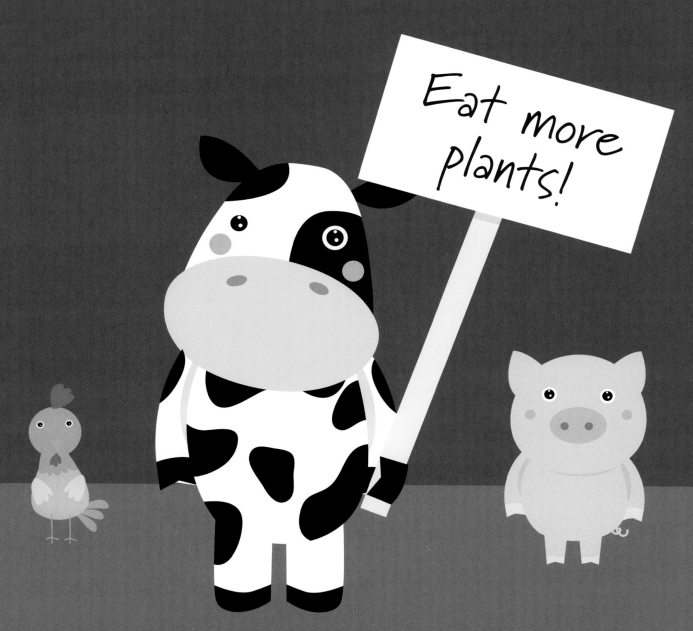

Meat is probably one of the most controversial foods. By now, you've probably already decided whether you're going to include meat in your diet or not. Either choice can lead to good health. Meat is a good source of complete protein, vitamins, and minerals. So are plants. People in many cultures live long, healthy lives with or without eating meat. If you do enjoy meat, a little can go a long way. Three to six ounces a day is plenty.

Small Habits

- ☐ **Enjoy fish weekly.** Enjoy fish once or twice a week. It is high in protein, has omega-3 fats, and has less saturated fat than meat.

- ☐ **Enjoy the entire egg.** Stop throwing the yolk out, and eat the entire egg. New research shows that whole eggs are not associated with heart disease.[20] This is great because the yolk contains the majority of the nutrients.

- ☐ **Flavor with meat.** Choose to serve dishes that use meat as a flavoring, not the main entrée, to reduce the amount of meat you eat.

- ☐ **Skip meat one day a week.** Pick a day of the week that you will not eat meat. This challenges you to expand your cooking repertoire to include more vegetables, beans, and grains.

- ☐ **Choose lean cuts.** Choose cuts of meat that are low in fat like chicken and turkey breast, pork loin, and lean beef steaks and roasts.

> Four out of the five longest living cultures in the world (Sardinia, Italy; Okinawa, Japan; Nicoya, Costa Rica; Icaria, Greece) eat mostly plants and eat meat sparingly. The fifth group (Seventh Day Adventists in Loma Linda, California) does not eat meat at all.[21]

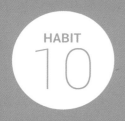

Enjoy dairy in moderation

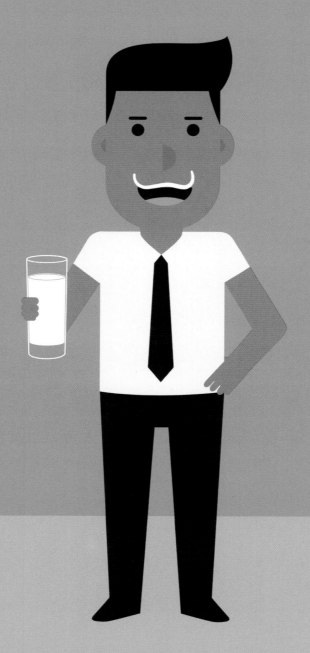

Most of us grew up being told to drink our milk to build strong bones. It is true that dairy products provide the nutrients necessary for good bone health, but don't despair if you're not a milk drinker. You can get those same nutrients from plants, specifically dark leafy greens. Still, nutrients alone aren't enough to build strong bones. You need sunshine and exercise, too. Sunshine is a much better source of vitamin D than milk, and exercise tells your body to absorb the nutrients.

Small Habits

☐ **Choose whole dairy products.** Choose whole (not reduced-fat) dairy products. New research shows that whole dairy products are not associated with heart disease.[22] This is good news because whole milk contains fat-soluble vitamins not found in skim milk.

☐ **Enjoy yogurt weekly.** Enjoy yogurt weekly or daily. The fermentation process that turns milk into creamy yogurt makes it easier to digest. Also, the beneficial bacteria in yogurt contribute to gut health, boost the immune system, increase nutrient absorption, and improve bowel regularity. Choose plain yogurt and sweeten with fruit.

☐ **Enjoy cheese.** Enjoy a small amount of cheese. The fermentation process used to create cheese unlocks nutrients, creates wonderful flavors, and makes it easier to digest.

Limit alcohol

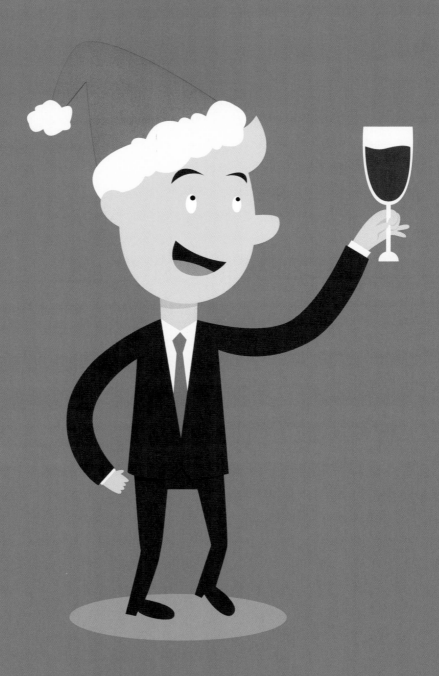

A little alcohol is fine (for most people), and it may even be good for you. The real problem with alcohol is excessive drinking, which may lead to unsafe driving, addiction, and disease.

If you decide to drink alcohol, here are some tips on how to do it safely. Drink with a meal, after you have begun eating, to slow down the absorption of alcohol into your bloodstream. Drink slowly because your liver can only process one serving of alcohol per hour. If you drink more quickly, excess alcohol builds up in your bloodstream, causing drunkenness.[23] Limit yourself to 2 drinks per day for males and 1 drink per day for females.[24]

Small Habits

☐ **Drink slowly.** Limit yourself to one serving of alcohol per hour, the rate at which your body can absorb alcohol.

☐ **Choose wine.** If you do include alcohol in your lifestyle, choose wine over beer and beer over spirits.[25]

☐ **Choose a substitute.** Instead of drinking alcohol, opt for nonalcoholic wine or beer, or drink sparkling mineral water and pure grape juice in a stemmed glass for festive occasions.

☐ **Forgo alcohol.** If you don't currently consume alcohol, do not start. The positives may not outweigh the negatives.[26] Focus on eating whole foods for longevity and enjoyment.

Serving Size	
Alcohol	Ounces
Beer	12
Wine	5
Spirits	0.5

Limit caffeine

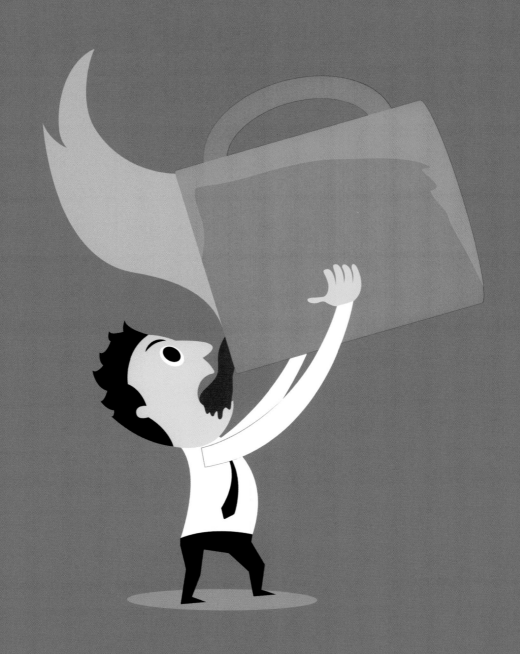

Who doesn't need a little boost to wake up from time to time? Caffeine can give you that boost, but its use is controversial. Some research says caffeine helps you focus and perform better in sports while other research says it makes you anxious and impacts your sleep. The reality is that caffeine affects everyone a little differently.

If you do decide to use caffeine, there are three things you should understand. First, caffeine does not actually give you energy. Rather, it blocks the messages from your brain that tell you that you are tired.[27] So, if you are using caffeine to mask a perpetual lack of sleep, the sleep deficit will catch up with you. (See *Habit 3: Sleep enough.*) Second, consuming 400 mg or more of caffeine daily can have negative health effects.[28] Third, the so-called "energizing" effects of caffeine will diminish with regular use, and you will eventually require more caffeine to "wake you up."

Beverage (8 fluid ounces)	Caffeine (mg)
Coffee brewed at home	100
Coffee-shop coffee	180
Espresso shot (1 fluid ounce)	60
Tea	40
Soda	40
Energy Drinks	80-240

Small Habits

- ☐ **Sip early.** Consume caffeine early in your day to maintain optimal sleep patterns at night.

- ☐ **Avoid coffee shops.** Choose home-brewed coffee over coffee-shop coffee. Coffee-shop coffee can have up to double the caffeine of the coffee you make at home.

- ☐ **Avoid cans.** Do not drink soda or energy drinks. They are generally unhealthy and are loaded with sugar and additives.

- ☐ **Drink decaf.** If you like the taste of coffee, drink decaf. It only contains 4-12 mg of caffeine per cup.

- ☐ **Choose tea.** Choose tea over coffee. It has much less caffeine than coffee, especially green tea.

- ☐ **Choose herbal tea.** Enjoy herbal tea instead of tea or coffee. Herbal tea has no caffeine and many types have medicinal properties.

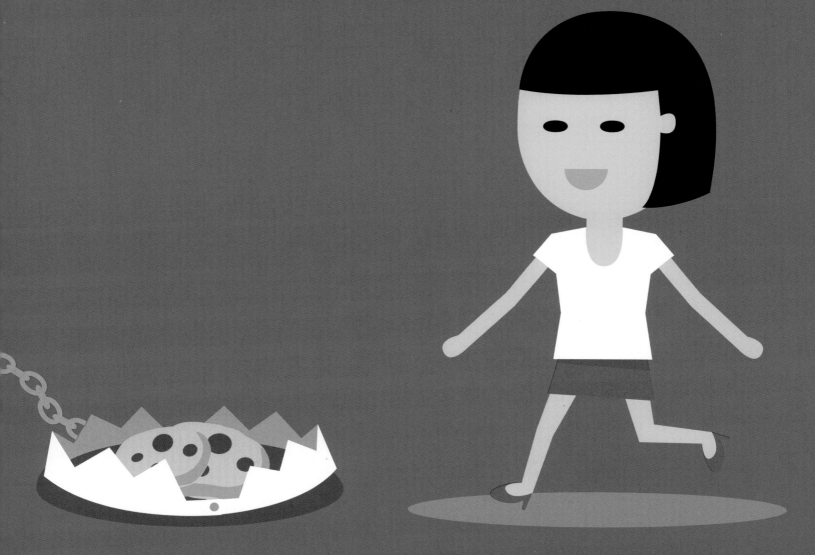

There's a lot of talk about sugar. Does it make you gain weight? Does it cause diabetes? Is it addictive? The answers to all these questions are not very clear. Sugar is not bad for you unless you eat too much, which is true for just about any food. So what's the big deal? In today's world, sugar is prevalent and it's very easy to eat too much. This can cause weight gain that may lead to other problems including obesity, diabetes, and heart disease.

So how much sugar should you eat? The World Health Organization recommends limiting sugar to 6 teaspoons (24 grams) a day or less ideally. This may sound like the go-ahead for eating sweets in moderation, but you can easily consume 6 teaspoons of sugar from seemingly unsweet foods. For example, a hamburger bun, ketchup, and unsweetened breakfast cereal each contain a teaspoon of sugar. While you may never turn down a piece of birthday cake, keep an eye on the amount of sugar in your daily diet.

Small Habits

- ☐ **Kick sugar out of your house.** Don't keep sugary foods in your home. Only invite sugar into your home for special occasions.

- ☐ **Avoid soda and fruit juice.** Avoid or limit soda and processed fruit juice (including products labeled 100% juice). They are almost pure sugar dissolved in water with little to no nutritional value.

- ☐ **Substitute fruit.** Eat fruit, nature's dessert, instead of sugary desserts. The flavors in fruit are delightful. Even though fruit contains sugar, the fiber in fruit slows down digestion, giving the body the time it needs to digest the sugar properly.

- ☐ **Enjoy dessert after a meal.** If you do eat dessert on occasion, eat it after a meal. That way the sugar is diluted by what you have already eaten, reducing the impact on your body.

- ☐ **Watch out for hidden sugar.** Check the label on packaged foods. Many contain much more sugar than you would expect (yogurt, granola bars, sports drinks, salad dressings).

- ☐ **Enjoy homemade soda.** If you aren't ready to give up soda entirely, substitute sparkling water mixed with 100% fruit juice.

Limit deep-fried foods

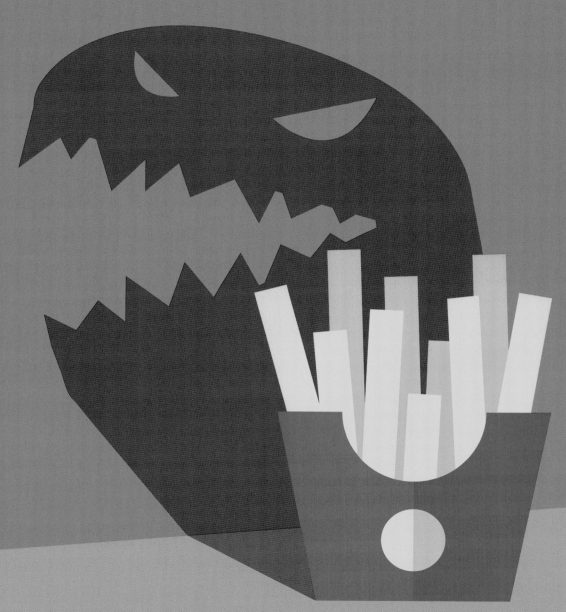

If you are like most people, you love eating french fries. It's no revelation that they're not the healthiest, but they're so good!

What's most important to understand about deep-fried foods is that deep frying adds a lot of calories. For example, a large baked potato has about 250 calories while the same potato made into french fries has about 800 calories. Another important thing to understand is that restaurants use cheap, low-quality fry oil that contains partially hydrogenated fat (trans fats), which is extremely bad for you, especially for your heart. So, even though you'll probably never give up deep-fried foods completely, go easy.

Small Habits

☐ **Avoid fried food at restaurants.** Be careful at restaurants. Many things that you might think are not fried, actually are. Restaurants fry most anything. If it's crispy, it's probably fried and contains twice the calories it would otherwise. Many restaurants can grill or bake foods upon request.

☐ **Avoid chips.** Go easy on chips. They are high in calories and salt and contain little nutritional value. Baked chips are a little better, but they also have a lot of calories with little nutritional value.

☐ **Avoid fried frozen foods.** Look out for frozen foods that have been previously fried (chicken strips, fish sticks, french fries). They have all the disadvantages of deep-fried food.

☐ **Avoid "baked" goods.** Watch out for "baked" goods that have been fried (donuts, cinnamon twists).

Forgo tobacco

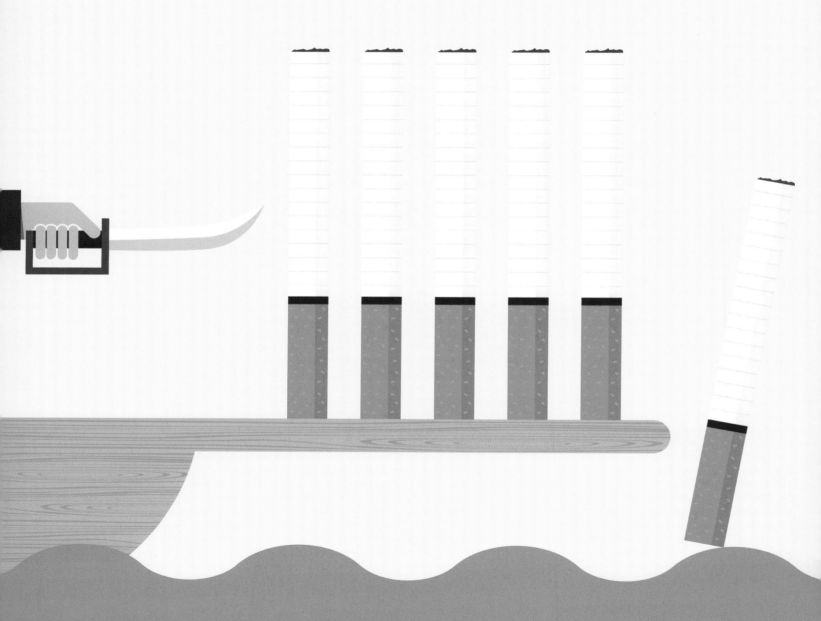

If you use tobacco, you already know it's really bad for you, and you've probably already tried to quit. All that remains to be said is that you can do it. You can quit. Maybe now is not the right time because of what you have going on in your life, but when the right time comes, you can do it. Each year over a million people are successful at quitting tobacco.[29] Most succeed within seven attempts.[30] You can succeed, too. Don't give up!

Small Habits

- ☐ **Give up one a week.** Give up one cigarette each week until you are tobacco-free. This will give your mind and body time to acclimate to the drop in nicotine.

- ☐ **Keep track.** Tally how many cigarettes you smoke each day and/or carry only the amount of cigarettes you intend to smoke for the day.

- ☐ **Smoke outside.** Don't smoke in your home or car.

- ☐ **Take a walk.** Replace a post-meal cigarette or smoking break with a short walk.

- ☐ **Ask for help.** Ask a friend to call you every day for support and accountability. Reach out to your friend when you need support.

- ☐ **Deep clean.** Clean your home (carpets, drapes, linens, floors) and cars. If you smell tobacco, you will subconsciously crave it.

- ☐ **Reroute.** Change your daily driving route to avoid the gas station where you buy cigarettes.

- ☐ **Learn while you commute.** Listen to an audiobook, podcast, or new music to stimulate your mind during your commute.

- ☐ **Calculate the cost.** Figure out how much money you will save by not using tobacco. Imagine what you could buy with the savings.

> **E-cigarettes**
> Electronic cigarettes are most likely less harmful than regular cigarettes. However, since they are not well regulated and are relatively new, the long-term effects are unknown.[31]

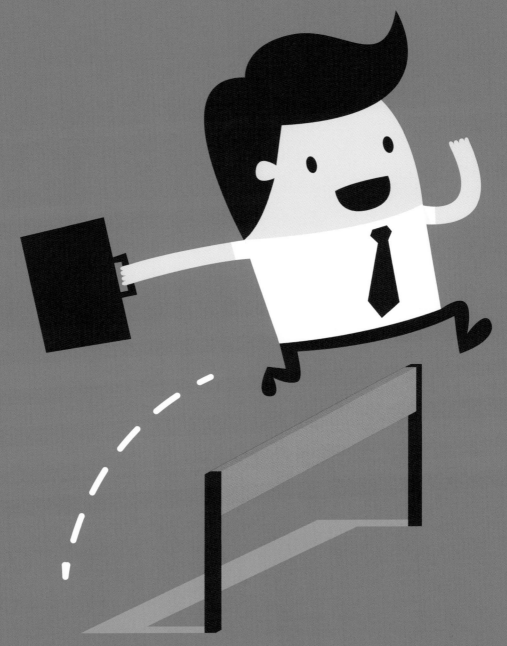

You know exercise is important, and you are likely already exercising in some way or another. The trick is finding the time and determination to do it over the long term. Think small and build from there. Remember this is something you need to do for the rest of your life, not just until you reach your target weight. Walk instead of drive. Mow the lawn. Take a walk at lunchtime. Every little bit helps.

Moving makes your heart and lungs stronger and more efficient, gives you more energy, helps you sleep better, and sharpens your mind. How much time you should move depends on how fast you move. If you do a light activity like walking, you should work up to 150 minutes a week. If you do an intense activity like running, you should work up to 60 minutes a week.[32] Ideally, you should spread your movement out over the week, but doing it all in one day works, too.

Small Habits

- ☐ **Start small.** If you don't enjoy exercising, begin with short walks to the end of your street or walking up and down the stairs. The distance will naturally increase over time.

- ☐ **Set yourself up for success.** If you plan to exercise in the morning, set out the clothes that you'll wear, your water bottle, and whatever you need the night before. This will not only be a visual nudge for you to exercise when the time comes, but it makes it easier to get moving.

- ☐ **Drink water.** Drink a glass of water before you work out and another after. If it's hot out or your workout is long, drink water during your workout.

- ☐ **Get outside.** Exercise outside to get the additional benefits of fresh air, sunshine, and an interesting environment.

- ☐ **Bring a friend.** Exercise with a friend. It can turn a hard workout into the highlight of your day.

- ☐ **Do it yourself.** Cancel your lawn service or maid service. Yardwork and housework are good ways to exercise.

Strengthen

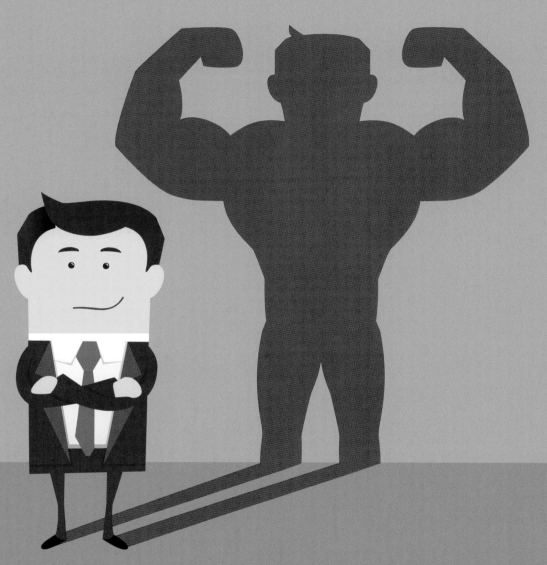

If strength training is your thing, enough said. Enjoy your workout. If you've never really been interested in strength training, read on.

Using your muscles does more than make you stronger and burn calories. It improves your coordination, reduces your chance of injury, improves your posture, and makes your bones stronger. Strengthening your muscles doesn't need to be difficult. You may already be doing it. Scrubbing the floor, washing your car, or doing yard work can be just as productive as going to the gym. However, if chores are not your thing, as little as 25 minutes per week of bodyweight exercises, resistance bands, or weights can work your muscles enough.[33]

Small Habits

☐ **Rest between workouts.** Let your muscles recover for 48 hours between intense workouts. If you like working out every day, alternate muscle groups or decrease the intensity of your workouts.

☐ **Start slowly.** When starting a strength-training program, train two days per week using moderate weights for healthy adults (light weights for older or frail adults). (American College of Sports Medicine)

☐ **Double dip.** Rotate muscle groups between sets so no rest is necessary and turn your strength workout into a cardio workout.

☐ **Maximize time.** Work more than one muscle group at the same time. Try pairing an upper body exercise with a lower body exercise (such as doing bicep curls while in a lunge).

☐ **Use bands.** Resistance bands are affordable, portable, and allow you to work the entire body.

Weight	Objective	Reps per set	Rest between sets
Light	Endurance and light strength	14-20 reps	20-60 seconds
Moderate	Endurance and strength	6-13 reps	1-2 minutes
Heavy	Strength	<6 reps	2-5 minutes

Source: American College of Sports Medicine.

Stretch

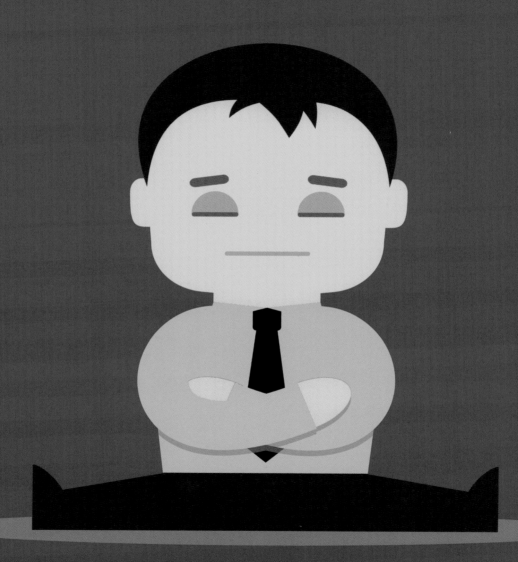

You may be thinking, "I don't have time to stretch. Is stretching even that important?" You're not alone. Most people don't stretch enough and think they're just fine without it, but stretching doesn't need to take extra time (and it is important). You can stretch effectively during a break at work, while you're on the phone, or while you wait in line at the store. Every little bit helps.

Regular stretching improves your flexibility and range of motion, making it easier to do everyday tasks. It helps prevent injury and improves your posture, which can alleviate back and neck pain. Stretching becomes even more important as you age and your body becomes less flexible. You only need to stretch 2-3 times each week to increase your flexibility.[34] Stretching more often will increase your flexibility even more.[35]

Small Habits

- [ ] **Warm up (dynamic stretching).** Gently mimic the movement of your workout to warm up your muscles (walk before running, rotate your arms before swimming, lift light weights before heavy weights).

- [ ] **Loosen up (static stretching).** Before workouts requiring flexibility (gymnastics, dancing, rowing), stretch specific muscles slowly, holding each stretch for 10-30 seconds and repeating 3-4 times.[36] It's best to warm up before doing this kind of stretch. Static stretches are also great after your workout or anytime for that matter.

- [ ] **Don't bounce (ballistic stretching).** Don't bounce when you stretch. Bouncing has limited benefit, can cause injury, and should only be performed when supervised by a professional.

- [ ] **Try yoga.** Attend a yoga class. Yoga is a great way to stretch your body, strengthen your body, and relax your mind all at the same time.

- [ ] **Stretch on the go.** Do simple stretches while standing in line at the store. Stretch your neck by tilting your head gently from side-to-side while sitting at a stop light.

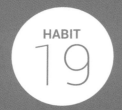

HABIT
19 Be positive

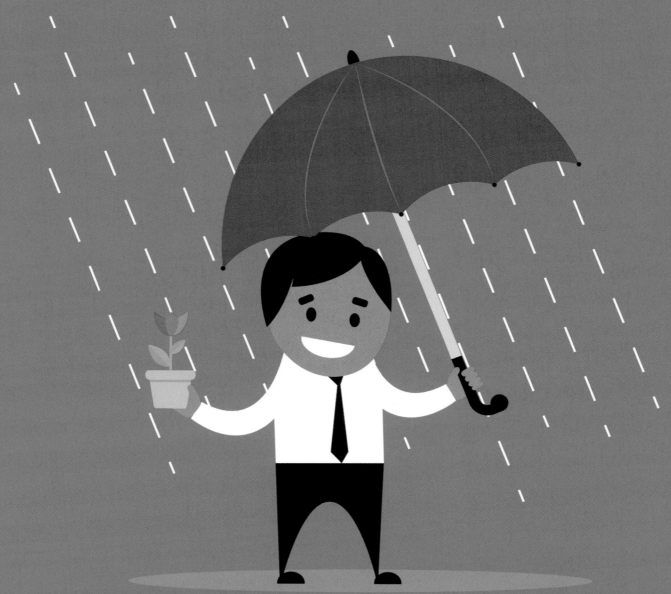

Some people seem to always be happy. Others rarely crack a smile. Based on your upbringing, your situation in life, and your genetic makeup, you're probably somewhere in between. Most people will never be the eternally happy person (in fact that person may not exist), but we can all become a little more positive with practice. Having a positive outlook on life can be as important for your health and longevity as exercising and eating right.[37]

Small Habits

- ☐ **Look on the bright side.** If something doesn't go your way, ask yourself what good might come of it.

- ☐ **Live in the present.** Make the most of every day by living as if today were your last day on earth.

- ☐ **Smile.** Wear a smile on your face. Smiling releases dopamine and serotonin in the brain, which makes us feel better. Also, smiles are contagious and can make everyone around you feel valued and good inside.

- ☐ **Keep good company.** Surround yourself with positive people to help elevate your mood.

- ☐ **Compliment others.** Always look for opportunities to give sincere compliments. By focusing on the good in others, the bad seems to fade away.

- ☐ **Thank others.** Recognize the positive things that other people do with a sincere "thank you." Both you and the person you thanked will feel better.

- ☐ **Avoid gossip.** Don't speak ill of others. Change the topic or excuse yourself if others are gossiping.

- ☐ **Be kind to yourself.** Don't say anything to yourself that you wouldn't say to a good friend. Counter any negative thoughts about yourself with encouragement and support.

- ☐ **Be grateful.** Make a list of things you are grateful for and come back to it on a rainy day.

Socialize daily

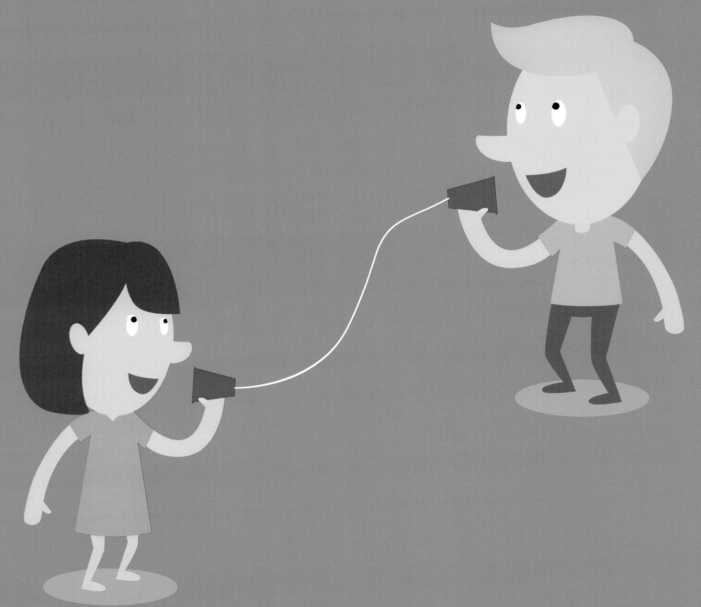

If talking with other people doesn't come naturally for you, becoming more social can be as daunting a task as giving up sugar. It's hard to know where to start or whether you want to start at all. It might be tough, but it will be worth it.

It may sound bizarre, but there are health benefits for socializing. When you get together with others, you usually end up laughing, which lowers your blood pressure and reduces stress hormones.[38] As a bonus, socializing improves your memory.[39]

Small Habits

- ☐ **Rekindle relationships.** Call an old friend or family member. Create a list of people to call or connect with and cycle through it every couple months.

- ☐ **Go deep.** Gather with people who care about you and can help you solve problems. It is important to be able to share personal information without worrying about being judged or betrayed. When it comes to socializing, quality is more important than quantity.

- ☐ **Make a friend.** Do something nice for someone, offer a compliment, or share some information and see how you connect. Spend time in the relationships that feel the most natural.

- ☐ **Schedule gatherings.** Set up a game night or movie night. Invite friends over for dinner.

- ☐ **Eat dinner together.** Talk about your experiences of the day as you enjoy dinner together as a family.

- ☐ **Seek out the lonely.** Spend time with others who might be lonely, like the new person at work, a shy person, or the elderly.

- ☐ **Serve.** Volunteering can be a great way to meet new people and develop relationships.

- ☐ **Take a class.** Take a class in yoga, cooking, or something else that interests you.

- ☐ **Listen.** Listen more than you speak and ask questions before you comment.

- ☐ **Talk it out.** When you are frustrated or have a problem, talk it out with a friend. Ideas will come as you verbalize your thoughts.

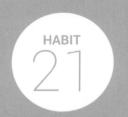

Recharge daily

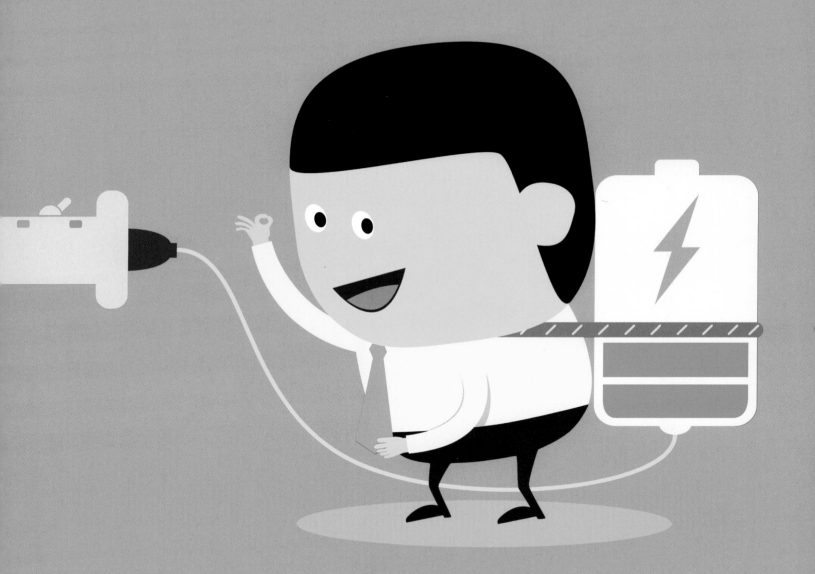

You're probably thinking, "Recharge? Right. I'll do that in between changing diapers and helping the kids with homework." But whether you realize it or not, you're probably already taking time to recharge. Watching your favorite TV show counts. Cooking a nice meal on the weekend counts. Reflecting while you exercise counts. When it comes to recharging, everyone does it differently. Think about what energizes you, and spend some time doing it each day. Consider upgrading your current recharging activities to ones that are even more satisfying.

When you are fully charged, you feel more positive emotions and interact better with others. You are more resilient when confronted with problems and can deal better with pain. Recharging lowers stress levels, which can strengthen your immune system and increase your lifespan.[40]

Small Habits

☐ **Reflect daily.** Set aside some time each day to be alone and meditate, pray, ponder, plan, journal, write letters, walk, or spend time in nature. When you reflect, you take time to consider what you are thankful for, what you have learned, and what you can do to change things for the better.

☐ **Create daily.** Try to develop an outlet like music, writing, dance, artwork, or gardening. Creating stimulates your mind and gives you a sense of identity.

☐ **Learn daily.** Whether you read a book, take a class, visit a museum, speak with an expert, or experience another culture, try to learn something new every day. Focus on things you care about. Develop an area of expertise. Learning will stimulate your mind and help you better understand your place in the world.

☐ **Play weekly.** Set aside some time each week to play a game, go on a picnic, hike, camp, cook, visit, watch a movie, or play a sport. Invite friends to join you or do it by yourself, whichever energizes or relaxes you more. Do something that you truly enjoy—something that is not part of your daily routine.

Recipicks

A "recipick" is a recipe for making your own recipe. Using a recipick is like ordering at a build-your-own burrito restaurant. You pick items from each row that suit your tastes. When you get to the last row, you're done!

RECIPICK
1

Vegetable Soup

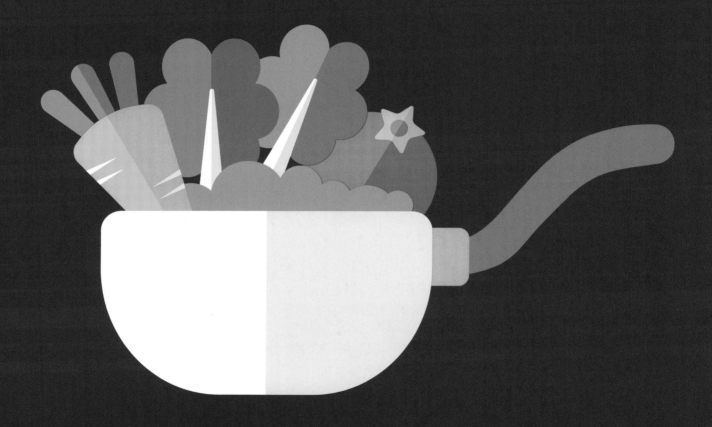

Vegetable soup is a great way to start any meal. It's delicious, nutritious, low in calories, and helps curb your appetite. It's also a great way to sneak in vegetables that you or your family would not normally eat.

Vegetables *6 cups*	• Onions • Garlic • Leeks • Parsnips • Turnips • Cabbage	• Broccoli • Cauliflower • Tomatoes • Carrots • Spinach • Celery	• Mushrooms • Potatoes • Zucchini • Kale • Corn
Oil *1 tablespoon*	• Butter • Olive oil		
Liquid *4 cups*	• Water • Vegetable broth • Chicken broth • Beef broth		
Herbs *Optional*	• Parsley, fresh • Cilantro, fresh • Mustard, fresh • Dill, fresh • 1 teaspoon basil	• 1 teaspoon oregano • 1 teaspoon thyme • 1 teaspoon cumin • Bay leaf	
Seasoning *Optional*	• Salt • Pepper • ⅛ teaspoon cayenne pepper • 2 tablespoons light cream, yogurt, or sour cream • 1-3 teaspoons lemon juice, lime juice, or balsamic vinegar		

Peel and dice vegetables. Heat liquid to boiling. In a separate pan, sauté vegetables in oil or butter on medium heat for 5-10 minutes, cover, and stir occasionally. Combine liquid, vegetables, and herbs. Simmer for 20 minutes. Optionally, liquify soup in blender and return to pan (remove bay leaf first). Add seasoning to taste.

Stir Fry

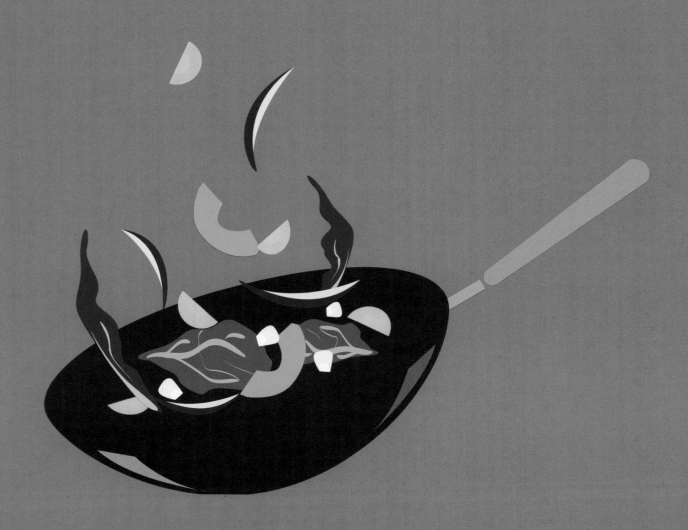

Stir fry is a great way to include lots of different vegetables in your meal. It can also be ready in minutes.

Vegetables *6 cups*	• Onions • Green onions • Garlic • Cabbage • Broccoli • Cauliflower	• Green beans • Carrots • Spinach • Bok choy • Celery • Mushrooms	• Sweet peppers • Hot peppers • Snow peas • Bean sprouts
Oil *1 tablespoon*	• Butter • Olive oil • Sesame oil • Peanut oil		
Protein *Optional*	• Beef • Chicken • Pork • Tofu • Shrimp		
Herbs *Optional*	• Parsley, fresh • Cilantro, fresh • Basil, fresh • Thyme, fresh • Mustard, fresh	• Mint, fresh • Sesame seeds • 1 teaspoon pressed ginger • ¼ teaspoon cayenne pepper	
Sauces *Optional*	• ½ cup teriyaki sauce • 1 tablespoon soy sauce • 1 tablespoon rice vinegar		

Sauté vegetables in oil on high heat, stirring constantly. Start with harder vegetables and protein. Don't overfill the pan. Cook 2 minutes, then add softer vegetables like broccoli and eggplant and sauces. Cook 2 minutes, then add greens and herbs. Cook 2 minutes more. Serve over rice.

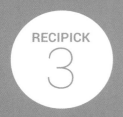

Fruit Salad

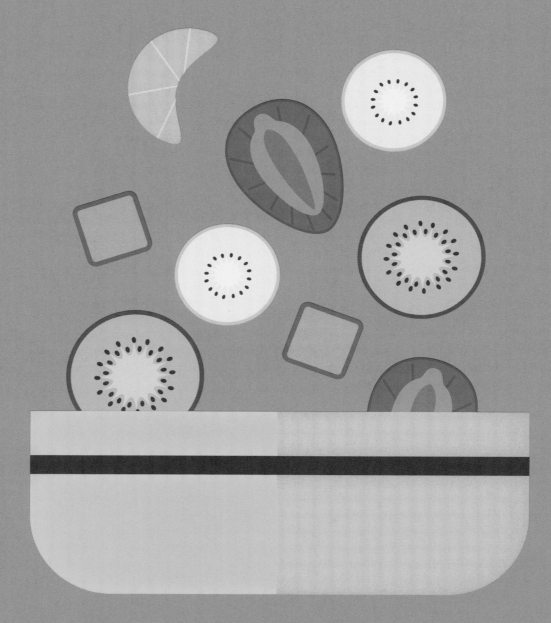

Fruit salad is light, sweet, and low in calories. Preparation only takes a few minutes, and the salad can be made differently every time depending on the fruits and ingredients that you choose, and what fruits are in season.

Fruits *6 cups*	• Blueberries • Strawberries • Pineapple • Bananas • Apples • Grapes • Kiwi	• Pears • Plums • Peaches • Oranges • Grapefruit • Mango • Melon
Sauce *Choose one*	**Creamy** • ½ cup plain yogurt • ¼ cup mayonnaise • 1 tablespoon lemon juice • 1 tablespoon honey • 1 teaspoon vanilla extract	**Clear** • ⅔ cup fresh orange or pineapple juice • ⅓ cup fresh lemon or lime juice
Accents *Optional*	• Toasted walnuts • Coconut flakes • Raisins • Poppy seeds • Black pepper	• Grated orange or lemon peel • Chopped fresh mint leaves • Shaved almonds • Dried cherries • Pine nuts

Prepare fruit and place in bowl. Prepare sauce with selected accents and stir into fruit.

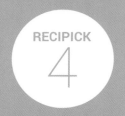

Smoothie

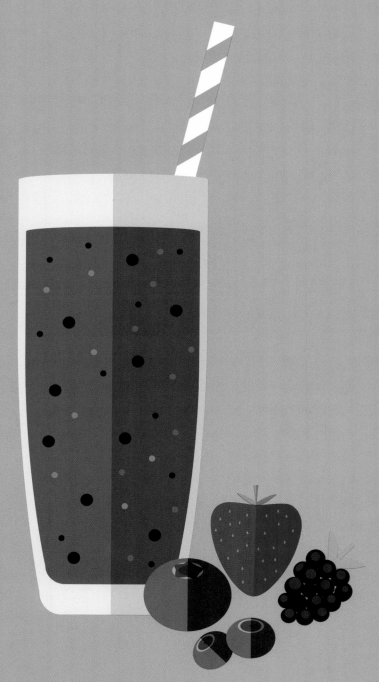

Smoothies are easy to make and quick to eat, and you can sneak in all sorts of healthy ingredients that normally might not appeal to you. You can whip up a nutritious and flavorful breakfast, snack, or dessert in no time!

Fruits *1 cup (fresh or frozen)*	• Blueberries • Strawberries • Pineapple • Bananas • Apples • Grapes • Kiwi	• Pears • Plums • Peaches • Oranges • Grapefruit • Mango • Melon
Vegetables *Optional*	• Spinach • Kale • Cabbage • Carrots	• Celery • Beets • Avocado
Liquid *1 cup*	• Plain yogurt • Fresh fruit juice • Milk (any kind)	• Coconut water • Water • Ice
Accents *Optional*	• 1 teaspoon vanilla extract • Honey • Flaked coconut • Fresh grated ginger • Ground flaxseed • Flaxseed oil	• Lemon juice • Cocoa • Protein powder • Nuts • Peanut butter

Combine fruits, vegetables, liquid, and accents in blender. Blend until smooth.

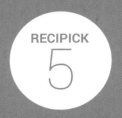

Beans and Rice

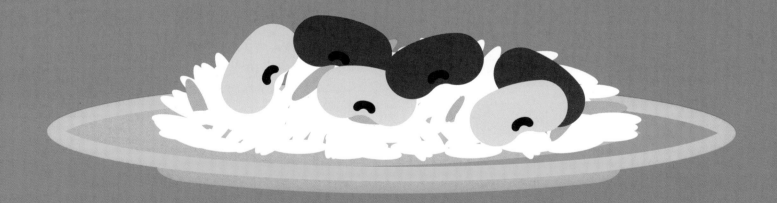

Beans and rice is inexpensive, satisfying, and provides a complete protein. Beans take awhile to cook, but you can shorten the time by using a pressure cooker or canned beans. Also, try freezing leftovers for a quick meal on another day.

Beans *4 cups (cooked)*	• Beans • Lentils
Vegetables *Optional*	• 1 cup chopped onion • ½ cup chopped celery • 8 ounce can tomato sauce • 1 cup chopped tomato
Meat *Optional*	• ½ pound chopped ham • ½ pound chopped smoked sausage • 1 ham bone
Seasoning *Optional*	• 3 cloves garlic, minced • ¼ cup chopped parsley • 2 bay leaves • 1 teaspoon Worcestershire sauce • Salt • Pepper • ¼ cup chopped cilantro • ½ teaspoon ground cumin

Sauté raw vegetables and meat in a large pot. Add remaining ingredients, cover with water, and cook until beans are soft and creamy (30-60 minutes). Smash some beans to make them creamier. Remove bay leaves and ham bone. Serve over rice. Optionally, add additional liquid and serve as a soup.

Bean Salad

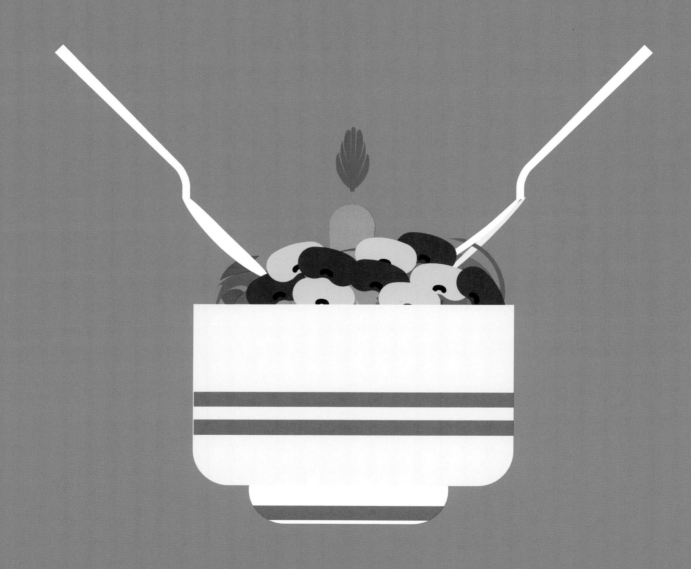

Bean salad is quick and easy to make and will last in the fridge for about a week. It's a great thing to have on hand to enhance any meal, or for a healthy, hearty snack.

Beans *2 cups (cooked)*	• Beans • Lentils

Salad Dressing *1/4 cup*	• Oil and vinegar • Oil and lemon or lime juice • Vinaigrette • Italian dressing • Russian dressing • French dressing

Vegetables *Optional*	• Garlic • Onions • Celery • Corn	• Avocado • Sweet peppers • Hot peppers • Tomatoes

Seasoning *Optional*	• Parsley • Cilantro • Rosemary • Thyme • Tarragon • Lavender	• Chives • Chili powder • 1 teaspoon salt • Black pepper • 1 tablespoon sugar • ¼ teaspoon ground cumin

Combine ingredients and toss.

Hummus

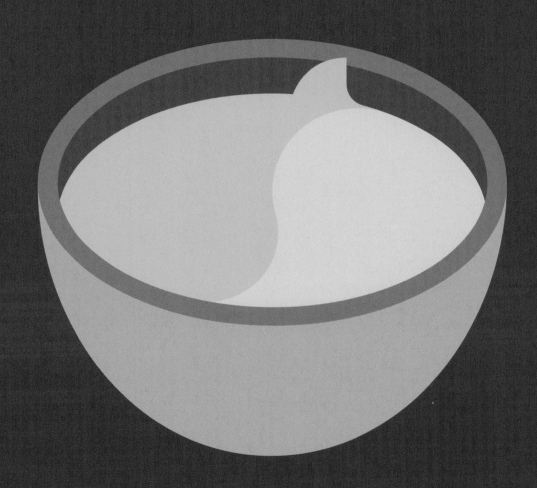

Hummus is a super healthy dip that you can make in minutes. Serve with fresh vegetables or pita bread. You can even spread it on sandwiches as a meat substitute.

Beans *4 cups (cooked)*	• Garbanzo beans • Black beans
Base *Include all*	• 2 cloves garlic, minced • ¼ cup extra virgin olive oil • 1½ teaspoons salt • 5 tablespoons lemon or lime juice • ⅓ cup tahini paste
Vegetables *Optional*	• Roasted red bell pepper • Roasted garlic • Spinach
Garnish *Optional*	• Sumac • Olives • Pine nuts • Extra virgin olive oil

Combine beans, base, and vegetables in food processor. Garnish before serving.

Vinaigrette

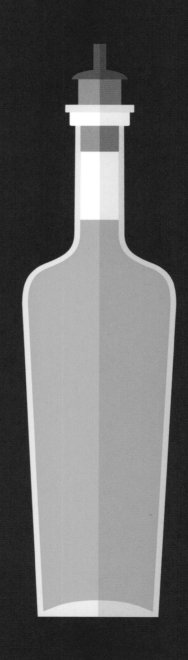

Vinaigrette is a light, flavorful dressing that can be used on almost any kind of salad. The flavor can be varied by using different types of vinegar, oils, and seasonings.

Vinegar *1/4 cup*	• Red wine vinegar • Balsamic vinegar • Lemon juice • Lime juice
Seasoning *Optional*	• ¾ teaspoon salt • 1 teaspoon sugar • 1 teaspoon honey • ¼ teaspoon black pepper • ¼ teaspoon crushed red pepper • 2 tablespoons Dijon mustard • 1 teaspoon garlic, minced • 2 teaspoons onions, minced • 1 tablespoon fresh herbs, minced • 1 tablespoon dried herbs • 1 teaspoon shallots, minced
Oil *1/2 cup*	• Olive oil • Walnut oil • Avocado oil • Canola oil

Mix vinegar and seasoning in a jar and shake well. Add oil. Shake well and serve.

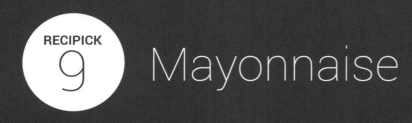

Mayonnaise

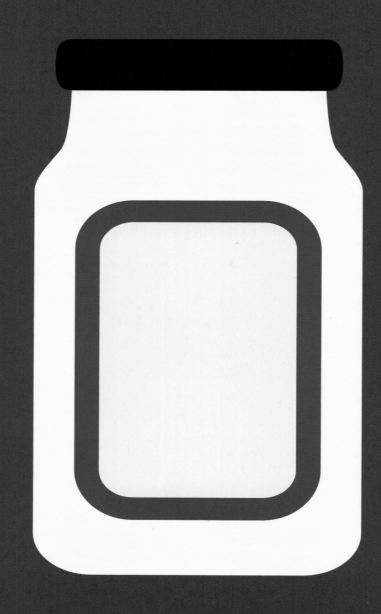

Making your own mayonnaise allows you to control the quality of the oil, and avoid mystery ingredients. Try adding different seasonings to make your own special sauce.

Base *Include all*	• 2 egg yolks or 1 whole egg (pasteurized) • 4 teaspoons vinegar or lemon juice • 1 teaspoon Dijon mustard • ½ teaspoon salt
Oil *1 cup*	• Olive oil • Walnut oil • Avocado oil • Canola oil
Seasoning *Optional*	• ⅛ teaspoon pepper • ¼ teaspoon sugar or honey • 2 cloves garlic, minced • 2 teaspoons finely chopped shallot • 1 tablespoon paprika • ¼ cup finely chopped fresh parsley, tarragon, or chives • 2 tablespoons finely chopped pickles • 2 tablespoons finely chopped olives • 2 tablespoons finely chopped vegetables • 1 roasted red pepper, minced • 1 teaspoon Louisiana-style hot sauce • 1 teaspoon Worcestershire sauce • 2 finely chopped capers • ¼ cup ketchup

In a glass bowl, briskly whisk together the base ingredients, then start adding the oil a few drops at a time until the liquid seems to thicken and lighten a bit. Slowly add the remaining oil as you continue to whisk. (A food processor or blender stick makes this job much easier.) Add seasoning. Refrigerate for up to 1 week.

Reviewers

Medical

Rahul Khare, MD, MS, FACEP
Dan Lonergan, MD
David Mitchell, MD, PhD

Nutrition

Veronica Niedzinski, MS, RD, LDN
Karen Schroeder, RD, LDN, HWC

Exercise

Michael Grimsley, MPH, CHES, CSCS

Psychology

Christian Laplante, PhD, R PSYCH, MFT

References

1. Greenberg J: Obesity and early mortality in the United States. *Obesity* 2013;21:405-412.

2. Grandjean A, Grandjean N: Dehydration and cognitive performance. *J Am Coll Nutr* 2007;26(5 Suppl):549S-554S.

3. Spigt M, Kuijper E, Schayck C, et al: Increasing the daily water intake for the prophylactic treatment of headache: A pilot trial. *Eur J Neurol* 2005;12:715-718.

4. Harrison Y, Horne J: The impact of sleep deprivation on decision making: A review. *Journal of Experimental Psychology: Applied* 2000;6:236-249.

5. Schmid S, Hallschmid M, Jauch-Chara K, et al: A single night of sleep deprivation increases ghrelin levels and feelings of hunger in normal-weight healthy men. *J Sleep Res* 2008;17:331-334.

6. Holzman D: What's in a color? The unique human health effects of blue light. *Environ Health Perspect* 2010;118:A22-A27.

7. Crispim C, Zimberg I, Dos Reis B, et al: Relationship between food intake and sleep pattern in healthy individuals. *J Clin Sleep Med* 2011;7:659-664.

8. Canene-Adams K, Lindshield B, Wang S, et al: Combinations of tomato and broccoli enhance antitumor activity in dunning r3327-h prostate adenocarcinomas. *Cancer Res* 2007;67:836-843.

9. Brown L, Rosner B, Willett W, et al: Cholesterol-lowering effects of dietary fiber: A meta-analysis. *Am J Clin Nutr* 1999;69:30-42.

10. Yang Y, Zhao L, Wu Q, et al: Association between dietary fiber and lower risk of all-cause mortality: A meta-analysis of cohort studies. *Am J Epidemiol* 2015;181:83-91.

11. Darmadi-Blackberry I, Wahlqvist M, Kouris-Blazos A, et al: Legumes: The most important dietary predictor of survival in older people of different ethnicities. *Asia Pac J Clin Nutr* 2004;132:217-220.

12. Liu, RH. 2004, *New finding may be key to ending confusion over link between fiber, colon cancer,* press release, 3 November, American Institute for Cancer Research, Washington, DC.

13. Grant W, Holick M: Benefits and requirements of vitamin D for optimal health: A review. *Altern Med Rev* 2005;10:94-111.

14. Milaneschi Y, Hoogendijk W, Lips P, et al: The association between low vitamin D and depressive disorders. *Mol Psychiatry* 2014;19:444-451.

15. Holick M: Vitamin D deficiency. *N Engl J Med* 2007;357:266-281.

16. Holick M, Chen T: Vitamin D deficiency: A worldwide problem with health consequences. *Am J Clin Nutr* 2008;87:1080S-1086S.

17. Ilahi M, Armas L, Heaney R: Pharmacokinetics of a single, large dose of cholecalciferol. *Am J Clin Nutr* 2008;87:688-691.

18. Norval M, Wulf HC: Does chronic sunscreen use reduce vitamin D production to insufficient levels? *Br J Dermatol* 2009;161:732-736.

19. Hunter J, Zhang J, Kris-Etherton P: Cardiovascular disease risk of dietary stearic acid compared with trans, other saturated, and unsaturated fatty acids: A systematic review. *Am J Clin Nutr* 2010;91:46-63.

20. Shin j, Xun P, Nakamura Y, et al: Egg consumption in relation to risk of cardiovascular disease and diabetes: A systematic review and meta-analysis. *Am J Clin Nutr* 2013;98:146-159.

21. Mishra B: Secret of Eternal Youth; Teaching from the Centenarian Hot Spots ("Blue Zones"). *Indian J Community Med* 2009;34:273-275.

22. Crichton G, Alkerwi A: Whole-fat dairy food intake is inversely associated with obesity prevalence: Findings from the Observations of Cardiovascular Risk Factors in Luxembourg study. *Nutr Res* 2014;34:936-943.

23. Lekskulchai V, Rattanawibool S: Blood alcohol concentrations after "one standard drink" in Thai healthy volunteers. *J Med Assoc Thai* 2007;90:1137-1142.

24. Camargo C Jr, Hennekens C, Gaziano J, et al: Prospective study of moderate alcohol consumption and mortality in US male physicians. *Arch Intern Med* 1997;157:79-85.

25. Di Castelnuovo A, Rotondo S, Iacoviello L, et al: Meta-analysis of wine and beer consumption in relation to vascular risk. *Circulation* 2002;105:2836-2844.

26. Semba R, Ferrucci, Bartali B, et al: Resveratrol levels and all-cause mortality in older community-dwelling adults. *JAMA Intern Med* 2014;174:1077-1084.

27. Persad L: Energy drinks and the neurophysiological impact of caffeine. *Neurosci* 2011;5:116.

28. Nawrot P, Jordan S, Eastwood J, et al: Effects of caffeine on human health. *Food Addit Contam* 2003;20:1-30.

29. Reitzes D, DePadilla L, Sterk C, et al: A symbolic interaction approach to cigarette smoking: Smoking frequency and the desire to quit smoking. *Sociol Focus* 2010;43:193-213.

30. Fiore M, Jaen C, Baker TB, et al: Treating tobacco use and dependence: 2008 Update. Clinical practice guideline. Rockville, MD: US Department of Health and Human Services. Public Health Service; 2008.

31. Farsalinos K, Polosa R: Safety evaluation and risk assessment of electronic cigarettes as tobacco cigarette substitutes: A systematic review. *Ther Adv Drug Saf* 2014;5:67-68.

32. Physical Activity Guidelines Advisory Committee (PAGAC). *Physical Activity Guidelines Advisory Committee Report*, 2008. Washington, DC, US Department of Health and Human Services, 2008.

33. Kim E, Dear A, Ferguson S, et al: Effects of 4 weeks of traditional resistance training vs. superslow strength training on early phase adaptations in strength, flexibility, and aerobic capacity in college-aged women. *J Strength Cond Res* 2011;25:3006-3013.

34. American College of Sports Medicine. Position Stand: Quantity and Quality of Exercise for Developing and Maintaining Cardiorespiratory, Musculoskeletal, and Neuromotor Fitness in Apparently Healthy Adults: Guidance for Prescribing Exercise. Retrieved from www.acsm.org.

35. Cipriani D, Terry M, Haines M, et al: Effect of stretch frequency and sex on the rate of gain and rate of loss in muscle flexibility during a hamstring-stretching program: A randomized single-blind longitudinal study. *J Strength Cond Res* 2012;26:2119-2129.

36. Robbins J, Scheuermann B: Varying amounts of acute static stretching and its effect on vertical jump performance. *J Strength Cond Res* 2008;22:781-786.

37. Danner D, Snowdon D, Friesen W: Positive emotions in early life and longevity: Findings from the nun study. *J Pers Soc Psychol* 2001;80:804-813.

38. Berk L, Tan S, Fry W, et al: Neuroendocrine and stress hormone changes during mirthful laughter. *Am J Med Sci* 1989;298:390-396.

39. Ybarra O, Burnstein E, Winkielman P, et al: Mental exercising through simple socializing: Social interaction promotes general cognitive functioning. *Per Soc Psychol Bull* 2008;34:248-259.

40. Segerstrom S, Miller G: Psychological stress and the human immune system: A meta-analytic study of 30 years of inquiry. *Psychol Bull* 2004;130:601-630.

Bloopers

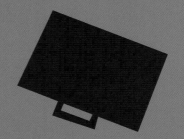
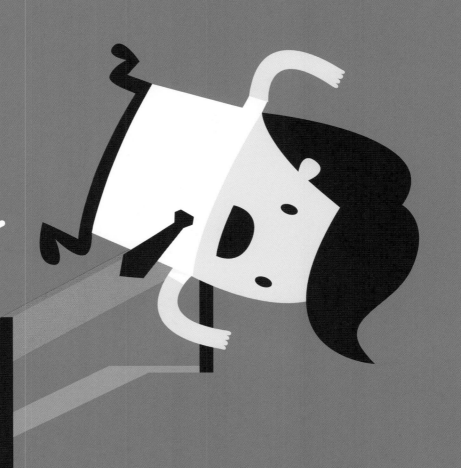

Limit sugar

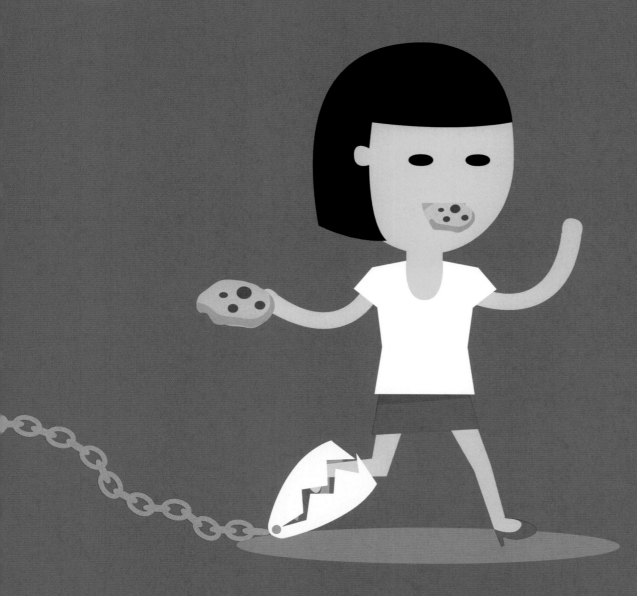

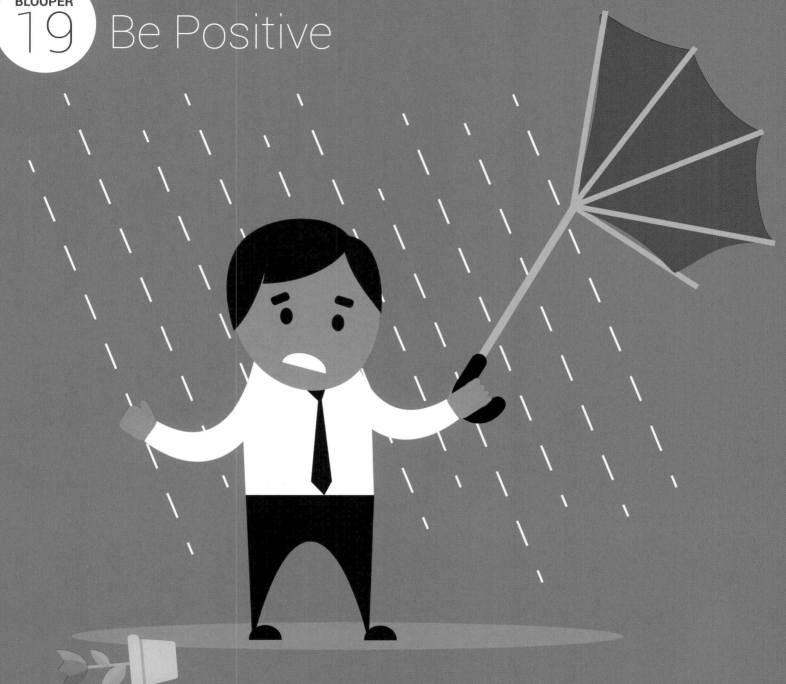

BLOOPER
19 Be Positive

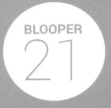

Recharge daily

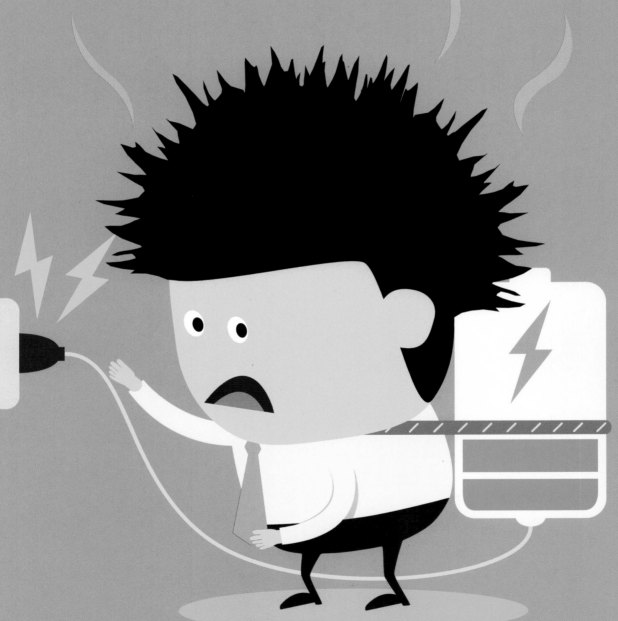

Enjoy sunshine in moderation

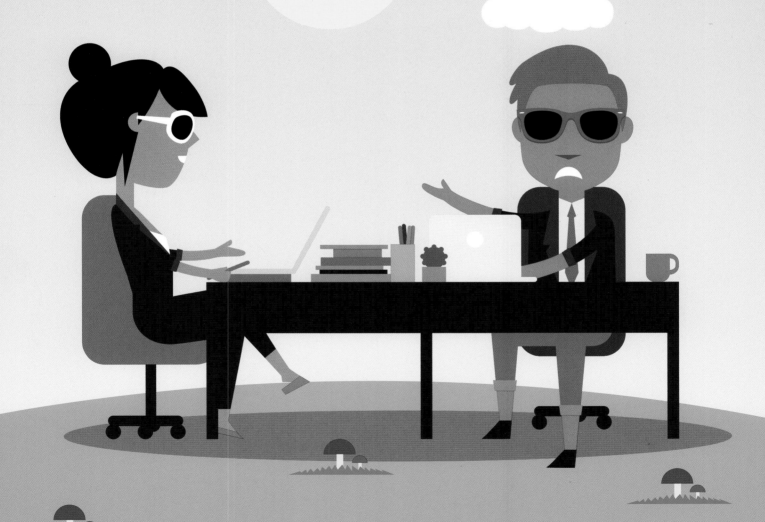

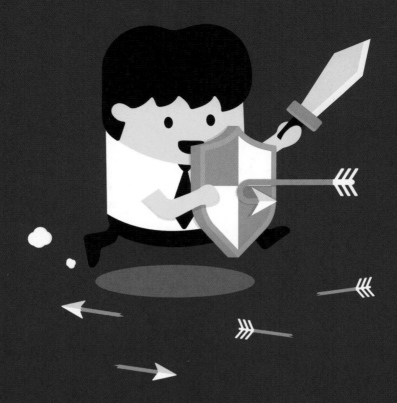

The Habit Gauntlet

Run the habit gauntlet before you start a new habit.

- ☐ **Step 1: Believe It.** Are you ready to do this habit for the rest of your life?
- ☐ **Step 2: Shrink It.** Can you make this habit any smaller?
- ☐ **Step 3: Trigger It.** What will trigger this habit?
- ☐ **Step 4: Prepare for It.** What can you do to prepare for this habit?
- ☐ **Step 5: Track It.** How will you track this habit?
- ☐ **Step 6: Be It.** What will help you do this habit for the rest of your life?